Simple English for J   als

すぐに使える
診療英語

加 藤 秀 一

Timothy M. Sullivan

南 山 堂

はじめに

　海外旅行で簡単な英語を話すだけなら，トラベル英会話の本があれば十分だと思います．しかしながら，仕事をするため，他国のことを深く学ぶためには英語の辞書を1冊覚えても足りないくらいです．私自身，かつては大学受験用の辞書で重要単語を覚えればおよそ大丈夫だと思っていたのですが……．

　とくに日本で英語を上達させるのはとても難しいですね．なぜなら，英語の上達には英会話の必要性と実際の英会話時間の両方が必要なのにもかかわらず，日本では多くの人にとってそのどちらも少ないからです．

　医療従事者の場合はどうでしょう？　近年，non-Japanese people が観光や仕事で来日しており，彼らが医療機関を訪れるケースが増えているので，よりいっそう英会話の必要性を感じている方も多いと思います．英会話を学ぶ時間はなかなかとれないと思いますが，医療という領域だけなら単語や表現の数は比較的限られているので，少ない時間で習得しやすいですよね．そこで，私が20年以上にわたって外来で使ってきた英語表現を本書にまとめました．

　医師や医学生は英語の医学専門用語はよく知っていますが，例えば日本人の患者さんに「これは癤です．」と言っても通じません．英語でも「This is a furuncle.」は一般的に通じないでしょう．「This is a boil.」ならわかってもらえます．「だるいですか？」は「Do you feel dull?」ではなく，「Do you feel tired [fatigued, sluggish]?」がよいでしょう．この本では，英語を話す一般の方が医療現場でどのように訴え質問してくるか，また，医療従事者がどのような英語で対応すればよいかがわかります．

　本書には下記の特長をもたせました．

① 専門用語の使用は極力避け，一般の英語表現を中心にした（主に米語表現）．
② 医療現場ですぐに使えるよう，role-playing 形式にはせず，場面ごとに適度な数のフレーズを選んで収載した．
③ 応用がきくシンプルなフレーズを提示するよう心がけた．
④ 1つの日本語表現に対し，なるべく複数の英語表現を提示できるよう努力した．
⑤ 受付から会計まで，医療機関における全過程を含めた．

　本書が医療の現場に接する医師・医学生，看護師・検査技師などの医療従事者，病院の受付担当者に活用していただけること，また一般の方々も含めて，旅行や留学で海外の医療機関を受診する場合にも役立つことを願っています．

2020 年 1 月

加 藤 秀 一

Contents

―――――――――― **本書中の記号について** ――――――――――

( ) 　例文中の（ ）は付加・省略可能な語，または補足を表す．

[ ] 　例文中の［ ］は直前の語または句と置換可能な語句を表す．
　　　句について置換開始箇所を明確にする必要がある場合には「 を
　　　用いて示した．

 参考・補足情報

 注意すべき発音

1 一般・電話対応

1-1 一　般

一般開業医

- a general practitioner

皮膚科［泌尿器科など］開業医

- a medical practitioner of dermatology [urology, etc.]

開業しています．

- I practice medicine.
- I have my own practice.
- I'm a practicing physician.

 physician は「内科医」を思い浮かべる方も多いかもしれませんが，いずれの診療科でも「医師」を意味します．

私は1999年に開業しました．

- I began practicing medicine in 1999.
- I've been in practice since 1999.
- I've been practicing medicine since 1999.

（医師が）診療する

- to examine [see] a patient

（患者が）〜について診察を受ける

- to consult [see] a doctor about 〜

加藤先生に〜（部位）を診察してもらう

- to have one's 〜 examined by Dr. Kato

健康診断を受ける

- to get [have] a physical (examination)
- to get [have] a medical checkup

✚ 専門医の名称など

診療所
 a (medical) clinic
 a medical office
 a doctor's office
 a health clinic
診察室
 an examination
 a consultation room
 a doctor's office
診療時間
 consultation hours
 office hours
診察券
 one's patient [patient's] card
 one's registration card
保険証
 one's health insurance card
初診料
 an initial-visit fee
再診料
 a revisit fee
 a follow-up visit fee
受付係
 a receptionist
担当医
 an attending doctor
内科医
 an internist

a doctor of internal medicine
 心臓専門医　a heart specialist,
  a cardiologist
 呼吸器専門医　a respiratory
  specialist, a pulmonologist,
  a chest physician
 消化器専門医　a gastrointesti-
  nal specialist
 神経内科医　a neurologist
 血液内科医　a hematologist
精神科医
 a psychiatrist
小児科医
 a pediatrician
 a children's doctor
外科医
 a surgeon
整形外科医
 an orthopedist
形成外科医
 a plastic surgeon
脳外科医
 a brain surgeon
 a neuro-surgeon
眼科医
 an ophthalmologist
 an eye doctor

耳鼻科医
- an ENT (doctor)
- an ears, nose and throat specialist
- an otolaryngologist

泌尿器科医
- a urologist

皮膚科医
- a dermatologist
- a skin doctor

婦人科医
- a gynecologist

産科医
- an obstetrician

麻酔科医
- an anesthesiologist
  - 麻酔担当医　an anesthetist

放射線科医
- a radiologist

口腔外科医
- an oral surgeon

1-2　電話対応

▶ 医師が電話に対応できない場合

加藤先生はいま患者さんを診ていて電話に出られません.

- **Doctor Kato is busy right now seeing patients.**

のちほど電話をかけ直してください.

- **Please call us again later.**
- **Please try calling us again later.**

先生は12:15もしくは6:15であれば都合がよいです.

- **He is available at 12:15 or 6:15.**

▶ 医師が電話対応できる場合

そのままお待ちください. 加藤先生と代わりますので.

- **Hold the line, please. I will put Dr. Kato on the phone.**

▶ 予約・診療時間の案内

このクリニックは予約できません．予約なしの患者さんのみ受け入れます．

- I'm sorry, we don't take appointments; we only take walk-in patients.

 You can't make an appointment with our doctor in this clinic. と言うと，相手に抑圧的になります．

受付時間は午前8：45〜12：00，午後2：45〜6：00ですが，火曜日・土曜日の午後と木曜日・日曜日は休みです．

- Our office hours are between 8:45 and 12:00 in the morning and (between) 2:45 and 6:00 in the afternoon. However, we are closed on Tuesday afternoon(s), Saturday afternoon(s), and all day Thursday(s) and Sunday(s).

予約制の場合

欧米では予約制が多いようです．

基本的にこのクリニックは予約制です．

- Basically, we take [accept] only patients who have made an appointment (in advance).
- I'm sorry, (unless it's an emergency,) we only take appointments.
- I'm sorry, we don't take walk-ins.
- You have to make an appointment if you want to see our doctor.
- You can see our doctor only by appointment.

いつがよろしいでしょうか？

- When would be convenient for you?

10月1日 午前10：00でいかがでしょうか？

- Would 10:00 a.m. on October 1st be convenient for you?

患者：はい，それでお願いします．

- Yes, that would be fine.

患者：いいえ，それは都合がわるいです．

- No, that is not convenient for me.
- No, that doesn't work for me.

繰り返します．10月1日 午前10:00です．

- Let me repeat the date and time. At 10:00 a.m. on October 1st.

▶ アクセスの案内

診療所は＿＿＿＿＿駅から歩いて6分のところにあります．

- Our office is (just) a six-minute walk from ＿＿＿＿＿ Station.
- It's a six-minute walk from ＿＿＿＿＿ Station to our office.

＿＿＿＿＿駅の南口を出てください．左手に「南口入り口」という名前の交差点が見えます．

- Proceed [Go] to the south exit at ＿＿＿＿＿ Station. There you'll see the "Minami-guchi Iriguchi" crossing [intersection] on the left.

その交差点を右に曲がって，500メートルほど歩きます．

- Turn right at that crossing and walk about 500 meters.

通りの右側に酒屋が見えてきます．

- You will see a liquor store on the right side of the street.
- Keep an eye out for a liquor store on the right side of the street.

そこは「旭町二丁目」という交差点のすぐ近くです．

- This is right near an intersection called "Asahi-cho Ni Chome."

そこから左手に私どものクリニックが見えてきます．

- If you look down the street to the left, you'll see our clinic.
- From there you can see our clinic down the street on the left.

2 〉受 付

2-1 初 診

▶ はじめに

すみません，私は英語が（あまり）わかりません．

- Sorry, I don't understand English (very well).

すみません，私はしっかりとは英語を聞きとることができません．

- Sorry, it's difficult for me to understand spoken English.
- Sorry, I don't quite follow you.
- Sorry, I'm not following you.

 この場合，Please speak slowly. と付け加えてもよいでしょう．

このクリニックは初めてですか？

- Is this your first time here?

▶ 保険と医療費

初診の場合，外国人向けの案内文書（Medical Fee Policy, p.153）を提示し，日本での医療費支払いの仕組みを理解してもらいましょう．

日本の健康保険に加入していますか？

- Do you have Japanese health insurance?

保険証を出していただけますか？

- Your health insurance card, please.

保険に加入している場合

保険に加入している場合は，日本では医療費をあなたと保険組合とで分担して負担します．

- If you have health insurance, you share the medical cost with your health insurance carrier [provider] in Japan.
- If you have health insurance, your medical cost is shared with your health insurance carrier [provider] in Japan.

あなたの負担金は医療費の10％から30％です．

- Your share will range from 10% to 30% of the total medical cost.
- You will be responsible「to pay [for paying] between 10% and 30% of your total medical cost.

加入しているが，今日は保険証がない

① 保険証を持参してこなかったのですか？

- Did you forget to bring your health insurance card?
- Did you forget your card (today)?

② 確認ですが，保険に加入したけれども，まだ保険証を受け取っていない，ということですか？

- Let me confirm: you have health insurance, but you didn't receive your card yet. Is that correct?

その場合（上記①か②の場合），今日は費用のすべてを支払ってください．次回，保険証を持っていらした際には，その費用の70％から90％をお返しします．

- In that case, you will have to pay all of your medical expenses today. But if you bring your health insurance card next time, we will refund you 70% to 90% of the expenses, depending on your policy.

後日の払い戻しについて

前回ここにいらした際に費用の100％をお支払いになりました．それは保険証を持参なされなかったからですが，今日は9月26日から有効の保険証をお持ちなので，費用の70％［90％］をお返しします．

- You paid 100% of the medical expenses on your last visit because you forgot to bring your health insurance card. Since you have your card today, and it is valid from September 26th, we'll refund you 70% [90%] of your previous payment.

保険に加入していない場合

保険に加入していない場合，診察のたびに医療費すべてを支払わなければなりません．

- If you're not insured, you will have to pay all of your medical expenses every time our doctor sees you.

先生が基本的な診察をして処方箋を書くだけなら，およそ3,500円くらいですが，血液検査をしたり，Ｘ線検査をしたりすると，10,000円以上になるかもしれません．およその額ですよ．医療費は検査によって変化します．薬の処方に際しては別途費用がかかるかもしれないのでご注意ください．

- If the doctor does a basic examination and writes a prescription, it will cost about 3,500 yen. But if you need a blood test or X-ray exam, it could cost over 10,000 yen. This is just a rough estimate. Medical expenses vary depending on the kind of examination. Please be aware that you might also have to pay additional charges for any medications prescribed.

トラベル保険に加入している場合

旅行者用の保険なら，診察のたびに医療費すべてを支払って，追って保険金を受け取ることができるでしょう．

- If you have traveler's health insurance, you will have to pay all of your medical expenses (upfront) every time you see the doctor. Your insurance company will reimburse you later.

健康診断のみの場合

単なる健康診断でお越しの場合，その費用は保険では支払うことができません．全部で12,000円以上かかります．

- If you are here only for a medical checkup, the expenses are not covered by health insurance. It will cost you over 12,000 yen.

どのような内容の健康診断をご希望ですか？

- What kind of medical check-up do you want (to have)?

通常の健康診断には肝機能や腎機能やコレステロールレベル，血球の数，心電図，胸部X線写真，尿検査が含まれます．

- A standard medical check-up includes liver function, renal function, cholesterol level, blood cell count, ECG, chest X-ray, and urine test.

そのほかに何か検査しておきたいことはありますか？

- Is there anything else you'd like to know?
- Is there anything else you need to have checked?

追加項目については追加料金がかかりますので，ご承知おきください．

- Please be aware that there is a surcharge for any additional items.

▶ 問診票の記入

問診票（Medical Questionnaire）p.154.

そちらに座り，問診票を記入して，名前が呼ばれるまでお待ちください．

- Please have a seat, fill out this form, and wait until your name is called.

✚ 頻度の高い既往症あるいは現病名

高血圧　high blood pressure	高尿酸血症　hyperuricemia
糖尿病　diabetes	痛風　gout
狭心症　angina (pectoris)	脳卒中　a stroke
心筋梗塞　myocardial infarction, a heart attack	アトピー性皮膚炎　atopic dermatitis, eczema
高コレステロール血症　high blood cholesterol	花粉症　hay fever, pollen allergy
高トリグリセリド血症　high blood triglyceride	

2-2　再　診

2回目ですか？

- Is this your second visit?

保険証と診察券を出していただけますか？

- Your health insurance and patient registration cards, please.

各月の最初の受診では，保険証と診察券の両方を見せてください．

- On the first visit of each month, you must show both your health insurance and patient registration cards.

その月の2回目の受診では，診察券のみ見せてください．

- On the second visit of the month, you only need to show your patient registration card.

3 診察の開始

3-1 呼び込みとあいさつ

（インターホンで）サリバンさん，中にお入りください.

- Mr. Sullivan, please come in.

サリバンさん，診察室3番にお入りください.

- Mr. Sullivan, please come into [to] room No.3.

おはよう. ／こんにちは. ／こんばんは.

- Good morning.／Good afternoon.／Good evening.

医師の加藤です.

- Hi, I'm Dr. Kato.

お座りください.

- Please take a seat.

今日はどうしました？

- What brings you here today?

 過去形を使った What brought you here?も，現在完了形の What has brought you here today?も問題ありませんが，上記の表現のほうが決まり文句です.

- What is your medical problem today?
- What is your issue today?
- What can I do for you (today)?

症状の経過を順番に説明してください.

- Please explain your symptoms in chronological order.
- Please explain your symptoms in the order that they occurred. Start with the first symptom…

3-2 患者さんからの訴え

~しづらいです.

- I have difficulty ~(drinking, eating, swallowing, speaking, remembering names, opening my mouth, standing up, seeing things, etc.).

この問題で昨夜は眠れませんでした.

- This problem kept me awake last night.

夜, 咳 [肩の痛み, 胸やけなど] で目が覚めます.

- My coughing [shoulder pain, heartburn, etc.] wakes me up at night.

できるだけ早くかぜを治したいのですが.

- I'd like to 「get rid of [get over] my cold as soon as possible.

痛み

背中が痛みます.

- My back hurts.
- I have back pain.
- I have a backache.

みぞおちが痛みます.

- I have pain in the pit of my stomach.
- The pit of my stomach hurts.

左の脇腹が痛みます.

- I have pain on the left side of my stomach.

左の脇の下が痛みます.

- I have pain in my left armpit.

胃 (おなか) が痛みます.

- My stomach hurts.

歯が痛みます.

- I have a toothache.

喉が痛みます.

- I have a sore throat.

喉が痛くて声が出せません.

- I can't speak because my throat is sore.

おなか［頭，首，背部など］が痛いです.

- I have a stomachache [headache, neckache, backache, etc.].

胸が痛みます.

- I feel pain in my chest.
- I have chest pain.
- My chest hurts.

胸の圧迫感を感じます.

- I feel pressure on my chest.

疲労感・全身衰弱

体がだるいです.

- I feel sluggish.
- I feel run-down.
- I feel tired.

月曜日から元気がありません.

- I have been unwell since Monday.

 unwell は British な表現.

- I have been feeling bad [sick] since Monday.

下肢がだるいです.

- My legs feel heavy.

寒気

（少し）寒気がします.
- I have [feel] a (slight) chill.
- I have the chills.

熱

熱があります.
- I have a fever [temperature].

まだ微熱があります.
- I still have a slight fever.
- I still feel slightly feverish.

37度くらいの微熱があります.
- I have a slight fever, around 37 degrees.

まだ39度の熱が出ています.
- I'm still running a fever of 39 degrees.

高熱が出ています.
- I am running a high fever [temperature].

高熱は出ていません.
- I don't have a high fever.

体温は昨晩下がりました.
- My temperature went down last night.

体温が38.5度まで上がりました.
- My temperature went up to 38.5 degrees.

体温が36.5度まで下がりました.
- My temperature went down to 36.5 degrees.

体温が2度下がりました.

- My temperature has gone down (by) 2 degrees.

咳

ひどい咳が出ます.

- I have a bad cough.
- I am coughing a lot.

咳で眠れませんでした.

- My cough is disturbing my sleep.
- My cough kept me awake [up] last night.

何度も咳払いをします.

- I clear my throat a lot.

痰

痰が喉にからみます.

- Phlegm sticks in my throat.
- I have phlegm in my throat.

痰が（たくさん）出ます.

- I'm coughing up (a lot of) phlegm.

息苦しさ

息苦しいです.

- I feel like I'm choking.
- I can hardly breathe.
- I'm out [short] of breath.

ときどき息切れがします.

- I sometimes run out of breath.

よだれ・つば

よだれが（たくさん）出ます.

- I'm drooling (a lot).
- I drool (a lot).

何度もつばを吐いています.

- I (have to) spit a lot.

いびき

昨晩，私がいびきをかいていたと妻が言っていました.

- My wife said I was snoring last night.

あくび

毎日あくびが（よく）出ます.

- I yawn (a lot) every day.

しゃっくり

しゃっくりが止まりません.

- I cannot stop hiccupping.

げっぷ

よくげっぷが出ます.

- I belch a lot.
- I burp a lot.

吐き気・嘔吐

吐き気がします.

- I feel like vomiting.
- I feel like throwing up.
- I am [feel] nauseated.
- I feel queasy.

- I feel sick to my stomach.

吐きました.

- I vomited.
- I threw up.

二日酔い

二日酔いです.

- I am hung over.
- I have a hangover.

便の性状

便が硬いです.

- My stool [poop] is hard.

 poop は「うんち」同様，主に子ども用語です.

- My feces are hard.

便がやわらかいです.

- My stool [poop] is soft [loose].
- My feces are soft [loose].

下痢

下痢をしています.

- I have loose bowels.
- I have loose bowel movements.
- My bowels are loose.

便秘

（ひどい）便秘です.

- I'm (really) constipated.

5日間便秘です.

- I've been constipated for the last 5 days.

旅行をするとき便秘になってしまいます.

- I get constipated when I travel.

腹部膨満

ガスが溜まっています.

- I have a lot of gas.
- I'm gassy.
- I feel gassy.

おなかが張っています.

- My stomach feels bloated.
- I feel bloated.

胸やけ・胃の具合

胸やけがします.

- I have heartburn.

胃が重苦しいです.

- I have a heavy feeling in my stomach.
- My stomach feels strange [weird, heavy].

胃の具合がわるいです.

- I have an upset stomach.

食べると胃がもたれます.

- Food sits heavy on my stomach.

睡眠障害

すぐに眠れません.

- I have difficulty falling asleep.

夜中に目が覚めてしまいます.

- I wake up in the middle of the night.

眠っていて目が覚めてしまうのです.

- I (often) wake up after falling asleep.

昨晩はほとんど眠れませんでした.

- I got (very) little sleep last night.
- I didn't sleep well last night.

昨晩は十分に睡眠をとりました.

- I got enough [plenty of, lots of] sleep last night.

毎晩よく眠れません.

- I'm not sleeping well every night.
- I have [am suffering from] insomnia.

睡眠不足です.

- I'm suffering from lack of sleep.
- I'm not getting enough sleep.

ずっと睡眠不足です.

- I have been suffering from lack of sleep.

この3日間, よく眠れていません.

- 「For the last three days [These past three days], I haven't been getting enough sleep.

記憶障害

忘れっぽくなりました.

- I've been forgetful.

頭がぼけてきました.

- I'm afraid I am becoming senile.

物忘れが多いです.

- I frequently forget things.

言語障害

言語障害があります.

- I have a speech impediment [disorder].
- I have difficulty speaking.

足がつる

左足がつりました.

- I had [got] a cramp in my left leg.
- I had [got] a charley horse in my left leg.

ふらつき

ときどき, ふらつきます.

- I sometimes have difficulty keeping [maintaining] my balance.
- I sometimes lose my balance.

めまい ⇒ p.135

3-3 問 診

～しづらいですか？

- Do you have difficulty doing～?
- Do you have any problems doing～?

 doing の例としては breathing, concentrating, swallowing, maintaining your balance, talking, reading, hearing what people are saying など.

いつからですか？

- Since when?
- When did your symptoms appear?

いつ気づきましたか？

- When did you notice the [this] problem?
- When did you notice your symptoms?

どのくらいその状態が続いているのですか？

- How long have you been feeling this way?
- How long have you been sick?
- How long have you been unwell?
- How long have you had these symptoms?

　患者：(今日で) 2，3日になります.

- (For) two or three days (now).

　患者：今週はほとんどです.

- For most of the week.

　患者：昨日からです.

- Since yesterday.

　患者：一昨日からです.

- It started the day before yesterday.

このことについて医師に診てもらいましたか？

- Did you see a doctor about this problem?
- Have you seen a doctor about this problem?

～(病名) と診断されたことがありますか？

- Have you ever been diagnosed with ～?

この問題で昨夜は眠れませんでしたか？

- Did this problem keep you awake last night?

市販薬を飲みましたか？

- Did you take any over-the-counter medicine?

患者：昨日，アセトアミノフェンを飲みました．

- I took Tylenol [Paracetamol] yesterday.

 Tylenol®，Paracetamol はそれぞれ米国，英国でごく一般的なアセトアミノフェン市販薬です．覚えておくとよいでしょう．

眼［皮膚，呼吸など］に問題ありますか？

- Do you have any problems with your eyes [skin, breathing, etc.]?
- Do you have any vision [skin, breathing, etc.] problems?

視覚［発声，聴覚，嗅覚，味覚など］は変化しましたか？

- Have you had any changes in your vision [voice, hearing, sense of smell, sense of taste, etc.]?

顔色がわるいですよ．

- You look pale.

痛み

まだ痛みますか？

- Are you still in pain?

どこが痛みますか？

- Where does it hurt?
- Where do you feel [have] pain?

ここは痛みますか？

- Does it hurt here?
- Is it sore here?

どのような痛みですか？

- What kind of pain do you have [feel]?

「痛み」の表現

鋭い痛み	a sharp pain	ヒリヒリする痛み	a stinging pain
鈍い痛み	a dull pain	キリキリする痛み	a piercing pain
ズキズキする痛み	a throbbing [pulsating] pain	割れるような痛み	a splitting pain
		しつこい痛み	a nagging [persistent] pain
刺すような痛み	a stabbing pain		
チクチクする痛み	a prickling pain		

痛みはどのくらい続きますか？

- How long does the pain last?

持続的ですか，それとも間欠的ですか？

- Is it continuous or intermittent?

空腹時痛ですか，それとも食後痛ですか？

- Do you feel pain on an empty stomach or after you eat?
- Do you feel pain before or after you eat?

かぜ・かぜ類似症状

頭痛や寒気以外に症状はありますか？

- Do you have any symptoms besides a headache and chills?

最近，かぜあるいはインフルエンザにかかった人をご存知ですか？

- Do you know anyone who caught a cold or the flu recently?

最近，かぜあるいはインフルエンザにかかった人と会いましたか？

- Have you recently come in [into] contact with anyone who caught a cold or the flu?

かぜをひいたような声をしていますね．

- Your voice sounds like you have a cold.
- You sound like you have a cold.

- You sound like you caught a cold.

喘息［インフルエンザなど］にかかったように思われます.

- It sounds like [as if] you (might) have asthma [the flu, etc.].

 会話では like のほうが一般的です.

熱

熱っぽいですか？

- Do you feel feverish?

家で体温を測りましたか？

- Did you take your temperature at home?

昨日の体温は何度でしたか？

- What was your temperature yesterday?

昨日はどのくらいの発熱でしたか？

- How high was your fever yesterday?

咳

（ひどい）咳は出ますか？

- Are you coughing (a lot)?
- Do you have a (severe) cough?

夜，咳で目が覚めますか？

- Does your coughing wake you up at night?
- Do you wake up because of your cough?

咳で眠れないことがありますか？

- Does your cough disturb [affect] your sleep?
- Is your cough disturbing your sleep?

痰

痰は出ますか？

- Are you coughing up phlegm?

痰の色は澄んでいますか，白っぽいですか，黄色っぽいですか？

- Is your phlegm clear, whitish or yellowish?

鼻水

鼻をすすっていますね.

- You are sniffling.
- You have the sniffles.

鼻水は出ますか？

- Is your nose running?
- Do you have a runny nose?

鼻水は水っぽいですか，それともねばねばしていますか？

- Is your nasal mucus watery or sticky?

鼻が詰まっていますか？

- Is your nose stuffy [congested, stuffed up]?
- Do you have 「a stuffy nose [nasal congestion]?

息苦しさ

何かするとき，息切れがしますか？

- Do you run out of breath when you do something?
- Are you short of breath when you exert yourself?
- Do you run out of breath easily?

いびき

いびきをかくと誰かに言われましたか？

- Did anyone mention [tell you] that you snore?
- Has anyone ever mentioned [told you] that you snore?

食欲

食欲はどうですか？

- How is your appetite?

嘔吐

吐きましたか？

- Did you vomit [throw up]?

便通

今朝は排便がありましたか？

- Did you have a bowel movement this morning?
- Did you empty [move, relieve] your bowels this morning?

今日はこの時間までに排便はありましたか？

- Have you had a bowel movement yet today?

この24時間の間に，何回排便しましたか？

- How many bowel movements did you have over the last 24 hours?

最後に排便したのはいつですか？

- When was your last bowel movement?
- What time was your last bowel movement?
- When did you last have a bowel movement?

規則正しく便通がありますか？

- Do you have regular bowel movements?
- Are your bowel movements regular?

下痢

下痢していますか？

- Do you have diarrhea [loose bowels]?

昨日は下痢をしましたか？

- Did you have loose bowels yesterday?

この24時間の間に，下痢で何回トイレに行きましたか？

- How many times did you have diarrhea [a loose bowel movement] in the last 24 hours?

便秘

便秘していますか？

- Are you constipated?

便秘傾向ですか？

- Are you often constipated?

何日，便秘していますか？

- How many days have you been constipated?

腹部膨満

おなかが張っていますか？

- Does your stomach feel bloated?
- Is your stomach bloated?

睡眠障害

昨日［昨夜］は何時に就寝しましたか？

- What time did you go to sleep yesterday [last night]?

昨晩はよく眠れましたか？

- Did you sleep well last night?
- Did you get a good night's sleep last night?

睡眠中に呼吸が止まると誰かに言われましたか？

- Did anyone mention [tell you] that you stop breathing in your sleep?
- Has anyone ever mentioned [told you] that you stop breathing in your sleep?

アレルギー

～にアレルギーはありますか？

- Are you allergic to ～?
- Do you have an allergy to ～?

犬や猫などのペットを飼っていますか？

- Do you have pets such as a dog or a cat?

花粉症はありますか？

- Are you allergic to pollen?
- Do you have a pollen allergy?

ストレス

ストレスは多いですか？

- Are you under much [a lot of] stress?
- Do you have a lot of stress?
- Are you stressed out?
- Do you have [feel] stress overload?

体重

体重はいくらですか？

- How much do you weigh?
- What is your weight?

患者：55kg です.

- I weigh 55 kilos [kilograms].

 kilos   [kíːloʊz]

体重は増えていますか？

- Are you gaining weight?
- Have you been gaining weight?

体重は減っていますか？

- Are you losing weight?
- Have you been losing weight?

体重は維持されていますか？

- Are you maintaining your weight?

めまい・その他の神経学的症状

めまいはしますか？

- Do you feel dizzy?

どのようなめまいですか？

- What is your dizziness like?
- Describe your dizziness.

部屋がグルグル回転しているように感じますか？

- Do you feel like the room is spinning (around)?

フワッとしますか？

- Do you feel like you are floating?

気を失いそうな感じですか？

- Do you feel faint?

首をひねったり，上を向くとめまいが生じますか？

- Do you feel dizzy when you turn your neck or look upward?

眼に異常はありますか？

- Do you have any visual problems?

手足の力が弱く感じますか？

- Do your hands, arms or legs feel weak?

そのとき意識を失いましたか？

- Did you faint at that time?
- Did you lose consciousness at that time?

最近，意識を失いましたか？

- Have you fainted recently?
- Have you lost consciousness recently?

どのくらいの時間，意識がなかったのですか？

- How long were you unconscious [out]?

発作

最後の喘息［心臓］発作はいつでしたか？

- When did you have your last asthma [heart] attack?
- When did you have your last episode?

1回の発作はどのくらいの時間続きますか？

- How long does each episode last?

手術・輸血

その病気［問題］で手術を受けましたか？

- Did you undergo [have] an operation for that disease [problem, issue]?
- Were you operated on for that?

どの病院で手術を受けたのですか？

- At which hospital did you undergo [have] the operation?
- Which hospital did you go to for the operation?
- Where did you have the operation done?

肺の手術を受けましたか？

- Did you have an operation on your lung?
- Did you have a lung operation?

誰があなたの肺がんの手術をしたのですか？

- Who operated on you for lung cancer?
- Who performed the operation on you for lung cancer?
- What doctor performed the procedure?

手術に際して輸血されましたか？

- Did you have a blood transfusion when you had your operation?
- Did you have a blood transfusion for your operation?

今までに輸血されたことがありますか？

- Have you ever had a blood transfusion?

3-4 問診（再診）

今日は気分はいかがですか？

- How do you feel today?

今日は元気ですか？

- Is your condition good today?
- Are you feeling good today?

すぐに回復しましたか？

- Did you recover quickly?
- Did you make a quick recovery?

すっかり回復しましたか？

- Have you completely recovered?

　患者：もうすっかり元気です．

- I'm quite well now.
- I'm feeling well now.

今日はとても元気そうです．

- You look much better today.
- You look good today.
- You look better than the last time I saw you.

腫れが引きましたね．

- The swelling has gone down.

（全身的に）よくなっていますか？

- Are you getting better?
- Are you starting to get better?
- Are you progressing nicely [well]?

　患者：よくなっているとは思えません.

- I don't seem to be getting (any) better.

（局所的に）よくなっていますか？

- Is your problem improving?

（局所的に）わるくなっていますか？

- Is your problem getting worse?

（局所的に）変わりはありませんか？

- Is your problem staying the same?

調子はいかがですか？

- How are you doing [feeling]?

　患者：咳が再発しました.

- My cough came back.
- My cough has returned.
- I'm coughing again.

　患者：リウマチが再発しました.

- I'm having a relapse [recurrence] of arthritis.
- I'm having another arthritis attack.
- My arthritis is「acting up [bothering me, flaring up] again.

　患者：心臓［喘息］の再発作が出ました.

- I had another heart [asthma] attack.

まだ何か症状がありますか？

- What symptoms do you still have?

まだ, だるいですか？

- Do you still feel tired [fatigued, listless, sluggish]?

体温は下がりましたか？

- Is your fever gone?
- Is your temperature back to normal?

咳 [かぜなど] は治りましたか？

- Did you get rid of your cough [cold, etc.]?
- Did you get over your cough [cold, etc.]?
- Is your cough [cold, etc.] gone?
- Are you over your cough [cold, etc.]?

薬はどのくらい残っていますか？

- How much medicine do you have left?
- How much medicine is left over?

薬をきらしましたか？

- Did you run out of medicine?
- Did you use up all your medicine?

耳鼻科の先生が処方した薬はきれていますか？

- Did you run out of the medicine your ENT (doctor) gave you?

3-5 診察手技

手

両手を差し出してください.

- Hold out your hands, please.

手の甲 [手のひら] を見せてください.

- Show me the backs [palms] of your hands.

体温

体温を測りましょう．この体温計を脇の下に入れてもらえますか？

・ **Let's take your temperature. Please put this thermometer under your arm.**

体温計は脇でしっかりとはさんでください．

・ **Please tuck this thermometer firmly under your arm.**

ピピッと音が鳴ったら出してください．

・ **You can take it out after it beeps.**

 it goes off という表現もあるが，銃・爆弾・警報・目覚まし時計など大きな音がする場合に用いるので，ここでは it beeps がよい．

✚ 部位の表現

腋窩（わき）　armpit(s), underarm(s)

乳房　breast(s)

臍（へそ）　navel

鼠径部　groin

腰骨（腸骨稜）　hip

殿部（しり）　buttocks, bottom, rear (end), behind, posterior

 尻の右側　the right side of your buttocks

大腿　thigh(s)

下腿　leg(s)

すね　shin(s)

ふくらはぎ　calf

 calf 　[kǽf]
複数形　calves 　[kǽvz]

手掌　the palm of the [your] hand

手背　the back of the [your] hand

足底　sole(s), the sole [bottom] of the [your] foot, the bottom of your right [⇔left] foot

足背　instep(s), the instep [top side] of the [your] foot, the top side of your right [⇔left] foot

	第1	第2	第3	第4	第5
手指	thumb	forefinger first finger index finger	middle finger second finger	ring finger third finger	little finger fourth finger
足趾	big toe	second toe	third toe	fourth toe	little toe

（体温を確認して）普通よりも高い［⇔低い］ですね.

- Your temperature is above [⇔below] normal.

眼

眼鏡を外してください.

- Please take off your glasses.

まっすぐ前を見てください.

- Please look straight ahead.

このペン先を目で追いかけてください.

- Please follow the top of this pen with your eyes.

かすんで見えますか?

- Is your vision blurry [cloudy]?

口腔

口を大きく開けて，アーと言ってください.

- Please open your mouth wide and say "aaah."

（口を開けたあと）一度，口を閉じて.

- You can close your mouth and take a (short) break.

（口を閉じたあと）また開けて.

- Please open it again.
- Please show me your throat again.

舌を出してください.

- Stick out your tongue, please.

扁桃腺が大きくなって，膿が出ています.

- Your tonsils are enlarged and covered with pus.

口中に潰瘍（アフタ）があります.

- You have a canker sore in your mouth.

- You have a mouth ulcer.

 舌圧子　a tongue depressor

胸部

胸の聴診をします．

- I'd like to listen to your chest.

シャツを上げてくれますか？

- Could you lift up your shirt, please?

シャツのボタンを外してくれますか？

- Could you unbutton your shirt, please?

深呼吸してください．

- Take deep breaths.
- Breathe deeply.

（深呼吸が不十分な場合）もっと大きく！

- Nice and deep!

（背部の聴診をするために）向こうを向いてください．

- Turn around and face the other way.
- Turn around and show me your back.

できるだけ速く，力強く息を吐いてください．

- Breath out as quickly and forcefully [strongly] as you can.

（服を脱いでいた場合）それでは，服を着ていいですよ．

- Okay, you can get dressed now.

シャツをズボンのなかに入れていいですよ．

- You can tuck in your shirt now.

シャツを下ろしていいですよ．

- You can pull down your shirt now.

頸部

首を診察させてください.

- Let me examine [check] your neck.

上2つのボタンをはずしてください.

- Please undo [unfasten] your top two buttons.

顎を上げてください.

- Please lift (up) your chin.

顎を下げてください.

- Please lower your chin.

少し下を見てください.

- Please look down a little [bit].

それでは, ボタンをかけていいですよ.

- Okay, you can button (up) your shirt now.
- Okay, you can fasten your buttons (now).

腹部

おなかを診察します.

- Let me examine your abdomen.

こちらに移動して, 仰向けになってください.

- Please move [come] over here and lie on your back.

靴を脱いでから診察台で横になってください.

- Please take off your shoes and lie (down) on the table.

ベルトを外してください.

- Please unfasten [loosen] your belt.

ズボン［スカート］を下げて, おなかを見せてください.

- Please「pull down [lower] your pants [skirt] to show me your abdomen.

膝を曲げてください.

- Put your knees up.
- Knees up.

どこが痛みますか？

- Where does it hurt?

（腹部を押しながら）ここは痛みますか？

- Is it sore here?
- Does it hurt here?

おなかが張っていると感じますか？

- Do you feel like your stomach is bloated?
- Do you feel bloated?

直腸

直腸を調べます.

- Let me examine your rectum.
- I am going to examine your rectum.

左側を下にして横になってください.

- Please lie on your left side.

下着を下げてください.

- Please pull down your underpants [male: shorts, female: panties].

肛門に指を入れます.

- I am going to insert my finger into your anus.

下肢

すねを診察させてください.

- Let me examine your shins.

足がむくんでいます.

- You have swelling in your legs.

• Your legs are swollen.

血圧・脈拍

血圧を測らせてください.

• Let's take your blood pressure.
• Let me take your blood pressure.

袖をまくってください.

• Roll up your sleeve.
• Pull up your sleeve.

血圧は120/80です.

• Your blood pressure is 120 over 80.

血圧が高いです.

• Your blood pressure is high.
• You have high blood pressure.

上の血圧が高いです.

• The top number is high.

下の血圧が高いです.

• The bottom number is high.

血圧が低いです.

• Your blood pressure is low.
• You have low blood pressure.

脈を測らせてください.

• Let's take your pulse.
• Let me take your pulse.

心拍数は70です.

• Your pulse rate is 70.
• Your heart rate is 70.

心拍数が高い［⇔低い］です.

- Your heart rate is high [⇔low].
- Your pulse rate is high [⇔low].
- Your pulse is quick [⇔slow].

脈が不整です.

- Your pulse is irregular.
- You have an irregular heartbeat.

4 身体測定

▶ 身長測定

身長は？

- How tall are you?
- What is your height?

　患者：I am 5 feet 8 inches tall.

身長を測りましょう．

- Let's measure your height.

靴を脱いでからここに立ってください．

- Please take off your shoes and stand here.

前方を見てください．

- Look ahead.
- Look to the front.

▶ 体重測定

体重はどのくらいですか？

- How much do you weigh?

　患者：I weigh 200 lbs.

 lbs 　[páʊndz]（ちなみに1 pound＝約454g）

I weigh 80 kilos [kilograms].

 kilos 　[kíːloʊz]

43

体重を測りましょう.

- Let's weigh you.

 家で自分の体重を計る　weigh oneself at home

"ゼロ"が表示されたら，体重計に乗ってください.

- Please step [get] on the scale when [after] it reads [says] "zero."

50kg です.

- You weigh 50 kg.

太りましたか？

- Have you gained weight?

痩せましたか？

- Have you lost weight?

▶ 腹囲測定

腹囲を測りましょう.

- Let's measure (the size of) your abdomen [stomach].
- Let's measure 「your abdominal circumference [the circumference of your abdomen].

5 視力検査

▶ 視力検査の説明

さあ，視力を測りましょう.

- Now(,) I'm going to test your eyesight [vision].
- Now(,) let's test your eyesight [vision].

この視力表で視力を測ります.

- Let's test your eyesight [vision] with this eye chart.

つま先を黄色のラインにあわせて立ってください.

- Please stand here with your toes on the yellow line.

この器具を使って左目を隠してください.

- Cover your left eye with this.

各リングの欠けている［開いている］部分がどこか答えてください.

- Please tell me where the missing [open] part of each ring is.
- Please locate the missing part of each ring.

　患者：上　top　　下　bottom　　左　left　　右　right　　左上　upper left　　右上　upper right　　左下　lower left　　右下　lower right

反対側を隠してください.

- Now(,) cover your other eye.

▶ 視力検査の結果

視力がいい［⇔わるい］です.

- You have good [⇔poor] eyesight.
- Your eyesight is good [⇔poor].

右目の視力は1.0です.

- Your right vision is 1.0.
- You have a visual acuity of 1.0 in your right eye.
- You have 1.0 vision in your right eye.

 英米では20/20(twenty twenty) や20/40と表現する.

6 血液検査

▶ 血液検査の説明・採血手技など

今日のところは診断がつけられません.

- I can't diagnose you today (because I don't have enough information).
- I don't have enough information to make a diagnosis today.

血液検査をしましたか？

- Did you have a blood sample taken?
- Did you get your blood tested?
- Did you have bloodwork done?

念のために血液検査をしましょう.

- To be on the safe side, let's check your blood.

何がわるいのか知るために血液検査をしましょう.

- Let me run [do] a blood test to see [find out]「what's going on [what the problem is, what's wrong with you].
- Let's do some bloodwork to see what's going on.

症状の原因を見つけるために血液検査をさせてください.

- Let me examine [check] your blood to find out the cause of your symptoms.

糖尿病［貧血など］なのかどうかを確かめるために血液検査をしましょう.

- Let me examine [check] your blood to see [find out] if you have diabetes [anemia, etc.].
- Let's do a blood test to check for diabetes [anemia, etc.].
- Let's test your blood for diabetes [anemia, etc.].

糖尿病［貧血など］の血液検査を受ける必要があります.

- **You need to get a blood test to check for diabetes [anemia, etc.].**

鉄量を調べるために，血液検査を受ける必要があります.

- **You need to get a blood test to check for your iron level.**

検査の日には朝食を抜いてください.

- **Please skip breakfast on the day of your examination.**

毎月［月に1回］，血液検査を受けなければなりません.

- **You should do a blood test「every month [once a month].**
- **You should have your blood examined every month.**

 have to は相手に強く響くので should のほうがよいでしょう.

他の異常を知りたいので，あなたの血液を再度調べるように検査会社に頼んでおきます.

- **I'll request the laboratory to examine your blood again for (any) other abnormalities.**
- **I'll have the lab check your blood again for (any) other abnormalities.**
- **I'll request the lab to run further testing on your blood sample to look for (any) other abnormalities.**

こちらに移動してください. 採血します.

- **Please come over here. I need to take a blood sample.**

握りこぶしを作っていただけますか？ ちょっと痛いですよ.

- **Please make a fist. You're going to feel a little sting [pinch].**

最後に食事あるいは飲み物を摂取したのは何時ですか？

- **What time did you last eat or drink something?**
- **When was the last time you ate or drank something?**

ここを指で2，3分圧迫してください.

- **Please apply pressure here with your fingers for a few minutes.**

結果は〜日にわかります.

- The results of your blood test will be available on 〜.
- We will get the results of your blood test on 〜.

ですから，10月3日以降に来てください.

- So please come back on the 3rd of October or any time after that.
- So please come back on October 3rd or any time after that.

何か大きな異常があった場合のみ電話します.

- I'll call you only if something major is wrong.
- I'll call you only if we find a major problem.
- I'll call you only if there's a major problem.

▶ 血液検査の結果

すべて正常です．健康体ですよ.

- Everything is normal [okay]. You are in good health.

血液に関してはまったく正常です.

- There is absolutely nothing wrong with your blood.

甲状腺に関する結果はまだ来ていませんが，その他はここにあります.

- I haven't yet received the results of your thyroid exam, but I have the rest of the results.
- I haven't yet received the results of your thyroid exam, but the other results are in.

結果はあなたが〜（疾患）であることを示しています.

- The results show that you have 〜.
- Judging from the results, you have 〜.
- Based on the results, you have 〜.

あなたの AST は30で，正常です.

- Your AST is 30, which is normal.

あなたの AST は高い［⇔低い］です．

- You have high [⇔low] AST.
- Your AST level is above [⇔below] normal.

あなたの AST は高く，それは肝機能に異常があるということです．

- You have high AST, which means your liver function is abnormal.

LDL-C の正常値は70～140です．

- The normal range of LDL-C is between 70 and 140.

UA の正常値は7以下です．

- A UA value below 7 is (considered) normal.

 A normal value of UA is below 7. という表現は自然ではありません．

この項目は肝機能の指標です．

- This (item) is an indicator of liver function.
- This (item) measures [indicates] liver function.

肝機能と腎機能はまったく正常です．

- Your liver and kidney functions are completely normal.

ナトリウム，カルシウム，糖はすべて正常です．

- Sodium, calcium, and glucose levels [readings, values] are all normal.

脱水症を疑う所見はありません．

- There are no signs of dehydration.
- The results show no sign of dehydration.

白血球が多い［⇔少ない］です．

- Your leukocyte count is high [⇔low].
- The number of leukocytes is abnormally [unusually] large [⇔small].

 前者のほうが普通の表現．

ＡとＢだけが少し異常でしたが，気にする必要はありません.

- Only A and B are slightly abnormal, but it's nothing to worry about.

この値は前回よりも低くなりました.

- This reading is lower than the previous one.

要するに，あなたは〜（疾患）だということです.

- The point is that you have 〜.

要するに［よいお知らせとしては］，あなたは〜（疾患）ではないということです.

- The point [good news] is that you don't have 〜.

以前やらなかった甲状腺機能の検査を追加しておきましたので，その分の代金1,000円を本日支払ってください.

- I ran some additional thyroid tests that weren't included in previous exams, so it will cost an extra 1,000 yen today.

その結果は数日後に私がチェックしておきます.

- I will check the results in a few days.

7 尿検査

▶ 尿検査の説明

尿を調べましょう.

- Let's get a urine sample.
- Let's test your urine.
- Let's do a urinalysis [urine test].

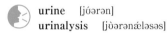
urine [júərən]
urinalysis [jùərənǽləsəs]

もし生理中なら，今回，尿検査は不要です.

- If you are menstruating, we don't have to do a urine test at this time.

待合室のトイレへ行って，このカップに尿を入れてください.

- Please go to the restroom in the waiting room and urinate into this cup.

初尿［中間尿］をカップの底から少なくとも2cmくらい入れてください.

- Please fill the cup with urine using the first [middle] part of your urine stream; fill it to at least 2 centimeters from the bottom.

手洗い場の近くに戸棚がありますから，そこにカップを置いてください.

- There is a built-in cabinet near the sink; please put the cup inside the cabinet.

排尿後はトイレからここに戻ってきてください.

- Please come back here after you're done.

排尿後は，医療費を支払って帰ることができます．

- After providing your urine sample, you can pay the receptionist, and you're free to go.
- After you provide a urine sample and pay the receptionist, you're free to go.

導尿による尿検査
正確な診断をするために，チューブを使って膀胱から尿をとります．

- For an accurate diagnosis, I need to drain [get] your urine directly from your bladder with a tube.

早朝尿検査
起床時最初の尿の中間を入れてください．カップのふちを折り曲げてから，尿を試験官に注ぎ入れて，その試験官をできるだけ早くこのクリニックへ持ってきてください．別の日にも同じことをしてください．

- First thing in the morning, please collect a mid-stream sample of your urine. To avoid spillage, squeeze the rim of the cup when you pour it into the test tube. Bring the sample to our office as soon as possible. Provide us another sample by doing this on a different day as well.

▶ 尿検査の結果

尿に関してはまったく正常です．

- There is absolutely nothing wrong with your urine.

尿が濁っています．

- Your urine is cloudy.

尿が濃い黄色です．

- Your urine is dark yellow.

尿検査では潜血が陽性と出ています．

- Your urinalysis indicated traces of blood.

尿検査で糖［タンパク］が出ています.

- Glucose [Protein] was detected on the urinalysis.
- There is glucose [protein] in your urine.

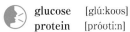
glucose   [glú:koʊs]
protein   [próʊti:n]

8 インフルエンザ検査

▶ インフルエンザ検査

インフルエンザの検査をさせてください.

- Let me run [give you] a flu test.
- Let's run a test to see if you have the flu.
- Let's test you for the flu.

 flu　[flúː]

サンプルをとるために，鼻にこのブラシを挿入します.

- I'll insert this brush into your nose to get [take] a sample.

少し痛いかもしれません.

- This might sting [hurt] a little bit.

少し不快かもしれません.

- You might feel a little discomfort.
- It's normal to feel some discomfort.

（検査中）頑張ってください（我慢してください）…

- Hang in there...

もう少しです，もう終わりですよ.

- Just a little bit more, we're almost done.

最終判定は5分後です.

- We'll know [have] the result in 5 minutes.

結果は陽性［⇔陰性］です.

- The result was positive [⇔negative].

 結果なので，過去形となります.

- You tested positive [⇔negative] for the flu.

 こちらのほうが普通の表現.

 インフルエンザ治療薬の服用法

（タミフル®）1回1カプセルを，朝食後と夕食後に今日から5日間飲んでください.

- Take one capsule after breakfast and (one after) dinner for five days starting today.

（リレンザ®）1回2ブリスター分の粉薬を，朝食後と夕食後に5日間吸入してください.

- For five days, inhale two blister doses of the powdered medicine after breakfast and dinner.

（イナビル®）一度に2キット分の粉薬を吸入してください.

- Inhale two kits of the powder medicine at one time.

（ゾフルーザ®）一度に2錠飲んでください.

- Take two tablets at once.

インフルエンザで学校や会社を休む期間の説明

日本では，インフルエンザに関する法律は学生だけに適用されます．

- In Japan, the law related to influenza is applied only to students.
- In Japan, the influenza law only applies to students.

しかしながら，現在ほとんどの会社もこのルールを採用しています．

- However, nowadays most companies follow this guideline as well.
- However, nowadays most companies adopt this policy as well.

学生さんは発症の次の日から5日間出席停止となります．

- (The policy states that) Infected students must be absent from school for five days excluding the day when their symptoms begin.

今回の場合，4月5日まで休み，つまり4月6日から学校に行けるようになります．

- In your case, you are required to stay away from school until April 5th. 「Which means [In other words,] you can go back to school on April 6th.

ただし，その出席停止期間中に熱のない日を2日含める必要があります．

- But you have to have two fever-free days during those days off.

熱がなかなか下がらず，予定の日までに熱のない日が2日ない場合，出席開始が遅れることになります．

- If you have a long-lasting fever and don't have two fever-free days before the scheduled date, then you have to postpone your return to school.

参考のため，これをお持ちください．

- Please take these guidelines for reference.

詳しくは学校［会社］に尋ねてください．

- For more [further] details, consult with your school [company].

9 ピロリ菌検査

ピロリ菌検査（尿素呼気試験法）

ピロリ菌は胃がんと関係があります.

- *Helicobacter pylori* is associated with gastric cancer.
- There is a correlation between *Helicobacter pylori* and gastric cancer.

袋を膨らますために息を吐くだけです. このテストは空腹で行います.

- To inflate the bag, you just need to breathe out. This test has to be done on an empty stomach.

ピロリ菌は飲んだ錠剤の主成分を変化させます.

- *H. Pylori* changes the main component of the medicine you take.

その菌はこの薬を変化させるのです. その変化した物質をあなたの呼気から検出できるのです.

- The bacterium will break down the medicine. The breakdown products can then be detected from your breath.

テストを終えるまでに約30分かかります.

- It takes about thirty minutes to complete the test.

まず, 袋を膨らませてください.

- First (of all), you inflate the bag.

次に, 薬を飲んでください.

- Second, you take the tablet.

20分後にもう一度, 袋を膨らませてもらいます.

- You have to inflate the bag again in 20 minutes.

結果は1週間で出ます.

- We'll have the results in a week.

ピロリ菌が検出されました.

- *H. pylori* was detected.

10 培養検査

培養検査のため，〜からサンプルをとらせてもらいます．

- Let me take a sample from your 〜 for a culture test.

結果は5日で出ます．

- We will get the results in five days.

検査では有意な細菌は検出されませんでした．

- No significant bacteria were detected on the test.

検査では〜菌が陽性でした．

- 〜 was detected on the test.

先日処方した抗生物質（抗菌薬）は検出された菌に有効です．

- The antibiotic I prescribed the other day can kill the detected bacteria.
- The antibiotic I prescribed the other day is effective against the detected bacteria.
- The antibiotic I prescribed the other day is effective against this particular bacteria.

 this particular bacteria はおかしいと思われた方へ．bacteria は bacterium の複数形ですが，会話やジャーナリズムにおいては例文のように単数扱いとなることがあるのです．Wall Street Journal でも This is caused by a bacteria borne by certain tiny ticks.というように使われているようです．

検出された菌は先日処方した抗生物質（抗菌薬）に感受性があります．

- The detected bacteria are sensitive to the antibiotic I prescribed the other day.

検出された菌は先日処方した抗生物質（抗菌薬）に耐性があります.

- The detected bacteria are resistant to the antibiotic I prescribed the other day.

胸部 X 線検査

▶ X 線撮影

その病院で胸の X 線写真を撮ってもらいましたか？

- Did you have [get] your chest X-rayed in that hospital?
- Did you have [get] an X-ray of your chest in that hospital?

その先生は X 線写真について何か異常があると言っていましたか？

- Did the doctor point out anything wrong with your X-rays?

胸の X 線検査をしましょう.

- I'd like to get [take] an X-ray of your chest.
- Let's get [take] an X-ray of your chest.
- Let's do a chest X-ray.
- I'm going to take an X-ray of your chest.
- I'd like to X-ray your chest.

X 線室へ移動してください.

- Please go to the X-ray room.
- The X-ray room is this way.

上着を脱いで, ピンクの検査着を着てください.

- Please remove your upper clothing and put on this pink smock.
- Please remove all upper clothing and change into this pink smock.

下着を着ていますか？ そうでしたら, シャツを脱いで下着だけになってください.

- Are you wearing an undershirt? If so, please take off your shirt. You can leave [keep] your undershirt [undergarments] on.

靴をはいたまま，ここに立ってください．

- Please stand here with your shoes on.

壁に向かってください．

- Please face the wall.

写真を撮るとき，「息を吸って止めて」と言います．

- When I take the X-ray, I'm going to ask you to inhale [breathe in] deeply and hold it.

大きく息を吸って，息を止めて．

- Inhale [Breathe in] deeply and hold it [your breath].

終わりです．普通に呼吸してください．

- We're finished [done]. You can breathe normally now.

服を着ていいですよ．

- You can put on your clothes now.
- You can get dressed now.

（フィルム現像の場合）現像中です．フィルムを現像するのに数分かかります．

- Development is 「under way [in progress]. It takes a few minutes to develop the film.

（デジタル撮影の場合）画像処理中です．すぐに画像を見ることができます．

- Imaging is under way. The image will be ready to see [read] in a moment.

▶ X 線検査の結果

X 線写真を読影します．

- I'm going to read [interpret] the X-ray for you.

X 線写真では異常ありません．

- This X-ray shows no abnormality.
- This X-ray is clear.

右の上のほうに異常な陰影があります.

* There is an abnormal shadow in the right upper field of this image.

胸部 X 線検査

12 CT/MRI 検査

▶ CT/MRI 撮影

更衣室で検査着に着替えてください.

- Please change into the exam wear [gown] in the locker room.

スリッパを脱いでからテーブルに横になってください.

- Please remove [take off] your slippers and lie on the table.

検査中は動かないでください. 15分くらいかかります.

- Please 「keep still [don't move] during the examination. It will take about 15 minutes to complete.

機械が大きな音をたてますので, 耳栓をつけてください.

- The machine is noisy [loud], so please wear these earplugs.

気分がわるくなったら, この緊急ボタンを押してください.

- If you feel sick [uncomfortable] during the exam, please [you can] push this emergency button.

▶ CT/MRI 検査の結果

これらの画像はあなたの頭部の横断面 [縦断面] を示しています.

- These images show cross [vertical] sections of your head.

出血 [梗塞, 腫瘍] はありません.

- There is no sign of bleeding [an infarction, a tumor].

肝臓に異常な陰影があります.

- There is an abnormal shadow on your liver.

大腸に憩室があります.

- You have a diverticulum in your colon.
- There is a diverticulum in your colon.

大腸　colon　[kóʊlən]
憩室　diverticulum　[dàɪvərtíkjələm]
憩室炎　diverticulitis　[dàɪvərtikjəláitəs]

憩室とは腸の壁におけるくぼみのことです.

- A diverticulum is a dent in the wall of the intestine.

大腸の壁の小さな袋 a small pouch of the colonic wall と説明することもできます.
たくさんの大腸憩室　many colonic diverticula

心配なものは何もありません.

- There is nothing to worry about.
- You have nothing to worry about.

70

13 心電図検査

▶ 心電図検査

次に，心電図をやりましょう．

- Next, let's take an ECG [electrocardiogram].

仰向けになってください．

- Please lie on your back.

看護師が心電図を担当します．

- The nurse will take it [your ECG].

最後に心電図をとってもらったのはいつですか？

- When did you last have an ECG (taken)?
- When did you last take an ECG?
- When was your last ECG?

異常を指摘されましたか？

- Did the doctor indicate [mention] that your ECG was abnormal?

シャツを上げてくれますか？

- Could you lift up your shirt(, please)?

シャツのボタンをはずしてくれますか？

- Could you unbutton your shirt(, please)?

腕時計をはずしてください．

- Please take off your wristwatch.

終わりです．

- We're finished [done].

x

服を着ていいですよ.

- You can put on your clothes now.
- You can get dressed now.

▶ 心電図検査の結果

心電図は正常です.

- Your ECG shows no abnormality.

心電図上, 不整脈を認めます.

- Your ECG detected an irregular pulse.
- Your ECG shows an irregular pulse [heart rate].
- There is an irregular pulse on your ECG.

この不整脈を治療する必要はありません.

- You don't need to get treatment for this.
- No treatment is necessary for this.

14 超音波検査

▶ 超音波検査

腹部の超音波検査をしていただきます.

- I would like you to get an ultrasound scan of your abdomen.

診察台に横になってください.

- Please lie down on the examination table.

シャツを上げて，おなかを調べますから.

- Lift up your shirt, I want to examine your abdomen.
- I want to examine your abdomen. Please lift up your shirt.

スカート［ズボン］を少し下げてください.

- Please「pull down [lower] your skirt [pants] a little.

両手は頭の下に置いてください.

- Put your hands under your head.

ゼリーをつけますので，冷たく感じます.

- I will put some gel on your abdomen; it will feel cold.

指示したら，息を大きく吸って止めてください.

- When I give the word, inhale deeply and hold it.

 the word は「指示，命令」の意味の場合，単数形となる.

息を止めたとき，できる限りおなかを突き出してください.

- When you hold your breath, stick out your stomach as forward [much] as possible.

やってみてください．それです．

- Give it a try. That's it.
- Try it. That's right.

（検査しながら）息を吸って，止めて！

- Inhale deeply and hold it!

普通に戻して．

- Okay, relax.

もう一度！

- Do it [the same thing] again!

終了です．

- (Okay,) We're done.
- (Okay,) It's over.

▶ 超音波検査の結果

この検査で異常はありません．

- There is nothing wrong according to this scan.
- This scan indicates no problems.

あなたの右の腎臓には直径5mm の結石［嚢胞］があります．

- You have a stone [cyst] 5 millimeters in diameter in your right kidney.

あなたの肝臓には嚢胞が2つあります．それぞれ直径20と35mm です．

- You have two cysts in [on] your liver. They are 20 and 35 millimeters in diameter, respectively.

15 胃内視鏡検査

▶ 胃内視鏡検査の事前説明

胃から出血している可能性があります.

- It's possible (that) it's gastric bleeding.
- It is likely that your stomach is bleeding.

その理由から, 胃カメラをするべきです.

- That's why you should get a gastroscopy.

土曜日に胃カメラを行っています.

- We do gastroscopies on Saturdays.

5月10日の朝8時でよろしいですか?

- Would 8:00 a.m. on the 10th of May be good for you?
- Would 8:00 a.m. on May 10th work for you?
- Would May 10th at 8:00 a.m. work for you?

胃を空にするため, 胃カメラの前日は夜中から何も飲食しないでください.

- Your stomach should be empty, so don't eat or drink anything after midnight on the day before the exam.

当日の朝は何も食べずに来てください.

- Please skip [don't eat] breakfast on the day of the exam. (That means no food, no drink.)

しかしながら, いつもの薬を少量の水で飲むのはかまいません.

- However, you can take your medicine with a small amount of water.

▶ 胃内視鏡検査

血液をさらさらにする薬は飲んでいますか？

- Are you taking any medication that would prevent your blood from coagulating?

検査ではファイバースコープを使います．喉をうまく通過させるために局所麻酔薬と鎮静剤を使います．

- We'll use a fiberscope to examine your stomach. To ensure the fiberscope smoothly passes through your throat, we'll numb it (first) with a local anesthetic and also give you a sedative.
- We'll have you swallow a fiberscope to examine your stomach. You won't feel discomfort since we numb your throat with a local anesthetic and also give you a sedative.

この氷をしゃぶって，ゆっくり溶かしてください．喉に麻酔がかかります．

- Put this (medicated) ice into your mouth and let it melt slowly; it will numb your throat.
- This ice is a local anesthetic. Let it melt in your mouth slowly. It will numb your throat.

この液体（消泡剤）を飲んでください．泡を抑えます．

- Please swallow this (liquid). It will suppress [prevent] bubbles from forming.

左下になってください．

- Please lie on your left side.

マウスピースをくわえてください．

- Hold this mouth piece in your mouth, please.

緊張していますか？

- Are you nervous?

リラックスしてください．

- Please relax.

76

胃カメラはもうすでに入っています.

- The scope is already in.

今からは嚥下しないでください.

- Please don't swallow anymore.

終わりましたよ.

- (Okay,) It's over.
- (Okay,) We're done.

胃の組織をいくつかとりましたので，病理学の先生に顕微鏡検査をしてもらいます.

- I took some tissue samples from your stomach. I will have a pathologist analyze them.
- I took some tissue samples from your stomach. We'll send them to pathology for (an) analysis.

結果は～日にわかります.

- We'll get the results of the biopsy on ～.
- We'll get the results from pathology on ～.

午前11時以後に飲み物をとることができます.

- You can drink something after 11:00 am.

午前12時以後に軽食をとることもできます.

- You can also have a light meal after 12:00 am.

午後1時まで車の運転はしないでください.

- Please don't drive until [before] 1:00 pm.

▶ 胃内視鏡検査の結果

組織検査の結果は悪性でした.

- The biopsy indicates [shows] malignancy.
- The biopsy indicates that the tumor is malignant.

組織検査の結果は良性でした.

- The biopsy indicates that the tumor is 「not malignant [benign].

 英語圏の人すべてが benign/benignancy という単語を知っ
ているわけではないので，良性をいう場合は，not malignant, no malignancy がよいでしょう.

胃に潰瘍［びらん，萎縮］を見つけました.

- I found 「an ulcer [erosion, atrophy] in your stomach.
- Gastroscopy indicated (that) you have an ulcer [erosion, atrophy] in your stomach.

16 診断・コメント

▶ 診　断

確定

〜と診断します.

- I've diagnosed your illness as 〜.
- My diagnosis is (that) you have 〜.

〜を患っています.

一過性の疾患や症状（時差ぼけ, 感冒など）の場合

- You are suffering from 〜.

慢性疾患（高血圧, 喘息など）の場合

- You have [suffer from] 〜.

（年単位など）長期の罹患を表現する場合

- You have been suffering from 〜.

間違いなく〜です.

- Definitely, you have got 〜.
- You definitely have 〜.

不確定

たぶん〜（病名）を患っているのでしょう.

- I think you have got 〜. （the flu など）
- I think you've got 〜.
- You seem to have 〜.
- I suspect you have 〜.
- It's likely (that) you have〜.

～かもしれないと考えています.

- I think you might have ～.

まだはっきりとしたことは言えないものの, ～かもしれません.

- It is too early to say, but you might have ～.
- It is too early to say for sure, but I suspect you might have ～.

訴えの多くは特徴がなく, 結論は出せません.

- Most of your symptoms are too general to draw a conclusion.

お聞かせいただいた限りでは診断が下せません.

- Based on what you told me (just now), I can't give you a diagnosis.
- Based on what you told me (just now), I can't diagnose you.
- Based on what you're telling me, I can't give you a diagnosis.
- I can't make an informed diagnosis based on the information you're providing.

さらなる情報がないと, この時点では診断が難しいです.

- It is very difficult for me to diagnose you at this time without more information.

▶ 病　因

患者：この病気の原因は何ですか？

- What causes this sickness [disease]?
- What is the cause of this sickness [disease]?

この病気の原因は不明です.

- The cause of this disease is unknown [not clear].
- We don't know what the cause is.

あなたの症状は〜から生じています.

- Your symptom is caused by 〜.

 〜に入る原因として overeating/eating too much/over-work/working too hard/working out too much/overexertion/lack of sleep/a cold/stress/dehydration/chemotherapy/radiation.

何かに感染したのだと思います.

- I think you have contracted [got] some kind of infection.

あなたの病気はあるウイルスによって起こります.

- Your disease is 「caused by [due to] a (certain) virus.
- This is a viral disease.

潜伏期は約2週間です.

- The latent period of this disease is about two weeks.

感染して2週間すると発症します.

- Symptoms appear about two weeks after you get infected.

この病気は伝染性です.

- This disease is infectious [contagious].
- This is a communicable disease.

この病気は飛沫感染で人から人へうつります.

- This disease can be passed [spread] from person to person by saliva.

あなたはおそらく彼からかぜをもらったのですね.

- You probably caught a cold from him.

あなたがそれを人にうつすかもしれません.

- You might spread it to others.
- You might infect somebody else (with it).

16

診断・コメント

マスクは感染症にかかるのを予防します.

- A mask helps prevent you from catching [getting] infectious diseases (from others).
- You can prevent catching infectious diseases with a mask.

マスクで感染症の拡散を防ぐことができます.

- You can prevent your spreading infectious diseases with a mask.

かぜをこじらせて肺炎になったのです.

- Your cold has developed into pneumonia.

雨で濡れるとひどいかぜをひきます.

- Getting wet in the rain can bring on a bad cold.
- Getting wet in the rain can lead to a bad cold.

はっきり言って, これは糖尿病と関係があります.

- Frankly, this problem is related to diabetes.

体内の抗体が甲状腺を攻撃するのです.

- Certain antibodies made in your body attack your thyroid.

疲れ・ストレスや夏の暑さからそのような症状が起きるのかもしれません.

- Your symptoms might (simply) be caused by fatigue, stress or the summer heat.

暑さ負けかもしれません.

- You might be suffering from the heat.
- You might be affected by the heat.
- The heat might be affecting you.

▶ 重症度

大したことはありませんが, ……

- It's nothing serious, but .....

状態は安定しています.

- You are in stable condition.

～の重症［中等症，軽症］例です.

- You have a severe [moderate, mild] case of ～.

 普通に考えると You <u>are</u> a mild case of hyperthyroidism. と表現するところだが，case は「病状」の意味としてこのように使われる. case の代わりに form も使うことができる.

重体です.

- You have a serious medical condition.

救急車を呼びます.

- I will call an ambulance for you.

早急に治療を必要とする問題ではないので，血液検査の結果を待ちましょう.

- This is not a matter that needs immediate attention [treatment]. Let's wait for the results of your blood test.

▶ 流行・症例数

麻疹が流行してきました.

- Measles has broken out.

今流行しています.

- There's a lot of it [this] going around.
- It is now peaking.
- It is now an epidemic.

 流行などの範囲を表す：全国的に all over the country, 局地的に locally.

わるいかぜが流行っています.

- There is a nasty cold going around.

流行がおさまってきています.

- It's subsiding (now).
- It's winding down (now).
- Peak season is over.

2型糖尿病（など非感染性疾患）が増えています.

- The number of people with type II diabetes is (greatly) increasing.
- The number of people with type II diabetes is approaching epidemic proportions.

17 治療方針・予後

▶ **治療方針**

内服薬

今日は薬は不要です.

- I will not prescribe you any medicine today.

薬を飲まずにこのまま様子をみてください.

- Let's wait and see how things go without any medicine.

痛み止めなしで自己管理できますか?

- Can you manage [make do] without (taking) a pain-killer?

薬で治るはずですよ.

- Medicine should [will] cure you.
- The medicine I am going to prescribe should [will] cure you.

この病気は治りませんが, 薬でコントロールできます.

- This disease is incurable, but it can be stabilized [controlled, managed] with medicine [medication].
- This disease can't be cured, but it can be managed with proper medication.

薬を飲んでこのまま様子をみてください.

- Let's see how things go with the medicine.
- Let's see how the medicine works.

5日分の薬を処方します.

- I will prescribe you (some) medicine for five days.
- I will prescribe you five days' worth of medicine.

17

治療方針・予後

85

抗生物質（抗菌薬）を使えば2～3日で熱は下がるでしょうが，7日間は飲むべきです．

- With the [this] antibiotic, your fever will be gone in a couple of days, but「make sure you [be sure to] take it for seven days.

しかしながら，必要に応じて解熱薬を使用してください．

- However, you can take an antipyretic「as necessary [if necessary, as needed].

点滴・注射など

抗生物質（抗菌薬）の点滴を受けたほうがよいでしょう．

- I strongly suggest we put you on an antibiotic IV [intravenous] drip.

栄養剤の点滴を受けたほうがよいでしょう．

- I recommend IV nutrition therapy.

抗生物質（抗菌薬）の点滴は経口に比べより効果的です．

- An antibiotic IV drip is more effective than taking it orally.

いままで点滴を受けたことがありますか？

- Have you ever had an IV drip?

3日間点滴を受ける必要があります．

- You need to undergo IV treatment for three days.

点滴をします．

- I will give you an IV (drip).

約1時間かかります．

- It will take about one [an] hour.

吐き気止めの注射をします．どちら側の腕がいいですか？

- I will give you「an injection [a shot] for your nausea. Which arm do you prefer?

浣腸をしますので，左下で横になって膝を胸に寄せてください．

- I will [am going to] give you an enema, so please lie on your left side with your knees pulled up toward your chest.

✚ 高血圧について

高血圧は脳卒中や心臓発作を引き起こす可能性があります．

- High blood pressure can lead to a stroke and [or] a heart attack.

寿命を延ばすには薬を飲むべきです．

- You should take medicine if you want to extend your life.
- This medicine will help extend your life.

薬を飲んで，血圧を下げましょう．

- Medication will help lower your blood pressure.
- You should take medicine to lower your blood pressure.
- I recommend you start taking blood-pressure medicine.

血圧をそれぞれ140，90未満に維持しましょう．

- Let's try to keep your blood pressures below 140 and 90 respectively.

今日から薬を飲んでください．

- You can [should] start taking the medicine today.

▶ 予 後

この病気は治ります．

- This disease is curable.
- This disease can be cured.

1週間くらいで治りますよ．

- You will get well in a week or so.

- You should be (feeling) better in a week or so.
- It will be a week or so before you 「get well [feel better].

治療なしで（自然に）治るでしょう.
- You should get better without any treatment.
- Your body will heal naturally without any treatment.

症状がよくならなければ，詳しい検査をします.
- If your condition doesn't improve, I'll do [give you] a (more) thorough examination.

長期の治療が必要です.
- You need long-term treatment.
- This requires long-term treatment.

この病気は治りにくい病気です.
- This disease is hard [tough] to 「recover from [get over].

これは命にかかわる問題です.
- This is [could be] a life-threatening problem [condition].
- This is a serious condition that could be life-threatening.

この病気は再発するかもしれません.
- This disease might recur [come back, flare up].
- You might have a recurrence [relapse] (of this disease).
- There is a chance of recurrence for this disease.

残念ながら，彼の病気は徐々に悪化するでしょう.
- I'm afraid his condition will gradually get worse.

残念ながら，しばらくの間，だるさが残るでしょう.
- I'm afraid you'll be feeling sluggish [weak, lethargic, under the weather] for a while.

毎年3,000人以上が～（例：気管支喘息）のために死亡します.
- Every year more than 3,000 people die of ～(ex. bronchial asthma).

18 休養・食事・運動の指導

▶ 休　養

十分に休息をとってください．

- You should [need to] get plenty of rest. Try to get plenty of rest.

2~3日の休養をおすすめします．

- I recommend a few days' rest.

できるだけ早く治すために2，3日休養したほうがよいでしょう．

- Taking a couple days off will help [accelerate, speed up] your recovery.

ゆっくり休んで水分をたくさん摂るようにしてください．

- Try to get some rest and drink lots of liquids [fluids].

ベッドでしっかりと休む必要があります．

- You need complete bed rest.

1日か2日，寝ていたほうがいいですね．

- I (highly) recommend (that) you stay in bed for a day or two.

たっぷり夏休みをとってください．

- I recommend you take a lot of time off this summer.

今日は学校を休んでいますか？

- Were you absent from school today?
- Did you take off from school today?

今日は仕事を休んでいますか？

- Are you off today?
- Is today your day off?

今日は仕事には行かず，一日中，寝ていたほうがよいでしょう．

- Today you should take the day off and stay in bed all day.

 the day off の the について：ここでは today という特定の日の話をしているので，a ではなく the がより自然な表現となります．

2〜3日，学校を休んだほうがよいでしょう．

- You should「take off from [stay away from] school for a few days.

2〜3日，仕事を休んだほうがよいでしょう．

- You should「take off from [stay away from] work for a few days.
- I strongly recommend you take off from work for a few days.

仕事を2，3日休んで疲れないようにしてください．

- Take a few days off from work and don't wear yourself out.
- Take off for a few days and don't over-exert yourself.

2〜3日で仕事［学校，通常］に戻れるはずです．

- You should be back to work [school, your normal routine] in a couple of days.

旅行は病状を悪化させます．

- Travel could [might] aggravate [worsen] your condition.

旅行は中止したほうがよいでしょう．

- I recommend you cancel [call off] your trip.
- It might be a good idea to cancel your trip.

▶ 食　事

食事に気をつかっていますか？

- Are you on a diet?

朝食は抜かないでください．

- You should not skip breakfast.

間食はしないようにしてください.

- You should avoid eating (snacks) between meals.

普通の食事に戻れるまでは，おかゆかそのようなやわらかい物を食べてください.

- I recommend (that) you eat 「rice gruel [soupy rice] or other soft foods until you can get back on a normal diet.

今は普通の固形のものは食べられないので，彼女にはおかゆかそのようなやわらかい物を食べさせてください.

- Since she can't eat normal solid foods right now, please give [feed] her rice gruel or similar soft foods.

1日のカロリー摂取を増やしてください.

- You should increase your calorie intake.

1日のカロリー摂取を控えめにしてください.

- You should reduce [decrease] your calorie intake.
- You should consume fewer calories per day.

1日どのくらいのカロリーを摂取するか計算してください.

- You should count how many calories you consume each day.
- You should count your calories on a daily basis.
- You should count your daily calorie intake.

1日1,500キロカロリーの摂取におさえてください.

- You should go [get] on a diet of 1,500 kilocalories a day.
- You should consume (no more than) 1,500 kilocalories a day.

高カロリーの食べ物は控えてください.

- You should avoid [refrain from, stay away from] high-calorie foods.

低カロリー食を守ってください.

- You should get on a low-calorie [low-cal] diet.

これはカロリーが高い.

- This is high in calories.

- This is a high-calorie food [dish].

これは200キロカロリーある.

- This has 200 kilocalories.
- There are 200 kilocalories in this.

薄味の食べ物が健康によいです.

- Lightly seasoned foods are healthier [better for your health].

塩分の多い食事は控えてください.

- Stay away from salty food.
- You should reduce [cut down on] the amount of salt [sodium] in your diet.
- You should get on a low-salt [low-sodium] diet.

あなたの場合，塩辛い食べ物は血圧を上げます.

- In your case, salty foods raise your blood pressure.

揚げ物は胃がもたれます.

- Fried food is [can be] heavy on your stomach.
- Fried food is hard to digest.

脂っこい食べ物は控えてください.

- You should avoid oily [greasy] foods.

甘いものや脂っこい食べ物は減らしてみましょう.

- Try to cut down on sweets and fatty foods.

脂っこい食べ物は血液中のコレステロール濃度を上げます.

- Greasy foods raise the cholesterol level in your blood.

動物性脂肪の摂りすぎです.

- You consume too much animal fat.

低脂肪食を守ってください.

- You should get on a low-fat diet.

しばらくの間，アルコールは控えてください．

- You should avoid [refrain from] drinking alcohol for a while.

長生きしたいなら，タバコは止めましょう．

- If you want to live longer, I recommend you stop [give up, quit] smoking.
- You will live longer if you stop [give up, quit] smoking.

チョコレートは止めること．

- Cut out chocolate.

果物はビタミンCが豊富です．

- Fruit is rich in vitamin C.

卵の黄身はコレステロールが多い．

- The yolk of an egg is rich [high] in cholesterol.

▶ 運　動

太りすぎです．

- You are overweight.
- You are not at a healthy weight.

体重に気をつけてください．

- You need to watch your weight.

体重計を持っていますか？

- Do you have a scale at home?

自分で（定期的に）体重を測定してください．

- Please weigh yourself (regularly).
- Please monitor your weight.
- Please keep an eye on your weight.

少し運動をすべきです．

- You should get some exercise.

運動と食事療法は病状を改善します.

- Exercise and diet will improve your condition.

定期的に体を動かしてください.

- You should exercise regularly.
- You need regular exercise.

スイミングはよい運動です.

- Swimming is good exercise.

ウォーキングを始めたほうがよいでしょう.

- You should start [take up] walking (for exercise).

✚ くすりの種類

処方薬　a prescription medicine [drug]

市販薬　an over-the-counter medicine [drug]

頓服薬　medicine only taken 「when needed [as needed]

漢方薬　Chinese herbal medicine

錠剤　a tablet

カプセル　a capsule

粉薬　powder [powdered] medicine

水薬　liquid medicine

トローチ　a medicinal candy, a lozenge

 medicinal [mədísənəl]

 （口中で）なめる　to suck on a lozenge

うがい薬　mouth wash, gargle

 この液でうがいする　to gargle with this solution

吸入薬　an inhalant

 inhalant [ɪnhéɪlənt]

点眼薬　eyedrops

 目薬をさす　to put drops in your eyes

点鼻薬　nasal spray medicine

外用薬　externally-applied medicine, an ointment

軟膏　sticky ointment

クリーム　cream-type ointment

湿布　a poultice

貼付剤（一般にいわれる湿布）　a medicated patch

坐薬　a suppository

浣腸液　an enema

かぜ薬　cold medicine

抗生物質（抗菌薬）　an antibiotic

抗ウイルス薬　an anti-viral medicine

解熱剤　an anti-pyretic, medicine for your fever

去痰薬　medicine for phlegm, medicine to loosen up your phlegm

咳止め　medicine for a cough, cough medicine

鼻水の薬　medicine for nasal drip

鼻づまりの薬　medicine for nasal congestion

抗ヒスタミン薬　an anti-histamine

炎症抑制薬　anti-inflammatory medicine

鎮痛薬　a pain-killer

かゆみ止め　anti-itch oral medicine

胃薬　medicine for gastric disorders

整腸薬　medicine for intestinal disorders	尿酸降下薬　an anti-hyperuricemic
消化薬　medicine for digestion	抗凝固薬　an anti-coagulant
制酸薬　an anti-acid, an antacid	抗うつ薬　an anti-depressant
吐き気止め　anti-nausea medicine	抗不安薬　an anti-anxiety medicine
胃の痙攣止め　medicine for stomach cramps	睡眠薬　a sleeping pill
緩下薬　a laxative	避妊薬　a birth control pill
降圧薬　an anti-hypertensive (medicine)	育毛薬　hair restoration medicine
コレステロール降下薬　an anti-cholesteremic (medicine)	水虫軟膏　anti-fungal ointment
	白癬内服薬　anti-fungal oral medicine
	かゆみ止めクリーム　anti-itch cream
	保湿剤　a moisturizer

▶ 内　服

お薬をお出しします.

- **I'll give you something [some medicine] (for this).**

ジェネリック医薬品を希望されますか?

- **Would you like generic medications?**

ジェネリック医薬品は先発品と同様に安全で効果があるとされています.

- **It is said that generic medications are as safe and effective as the brand-name products.**

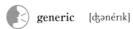 generic　[ʤənérɪk]

A のほうが B よりも効きます.

- **A works better than B.**

薬はすべて処方通りに飲みきってください.

- **You must take all the medicine as prescribed.**

このまま数日間，薬が効くか様子をみましょう.

- Let's wait for a few days to see how the medicine works.
- Let's wait for a few days to see how effective the medicine is.
- Let's wait for a few days to see if this medicine helps (improve your condition).

この薬はすぐには効きません. 2〜3日かかります.

- This medicine won't take effect right away; it will take a couple (of) days.
- You will feel the effects of this medicine in a couple days.

隣の薬局で処方箋の薬を出してもらえます.

- You can get the prescription filled in the pharmacy next to this clinic.
- The pharmacy next door will [can] fill your prescriptions.

どこの薬局でも処方薬を調合してもらえます.

- You can have the prescription filled at any pharmacy.

薬をもらって，すぐに休んでください.

- Get this prescription filled and go straight to bed.

1日1回服用してください.

- Please take it [this] once a day.
  - 朝食後に　　after breakfast
  - 昼食後に　　after lunch
  - 夕食後に　　after dinner
  - 寝る前に　　before bed, before bedtime, before you go to bed

1日2回服用してください.

- Please take it twice a day [twice daily].
  - 朝食後と夕食後に　　after breakfast and (also) after dinner
  - 朝食後と寝る前に　　after breakfast and before bed
  - 食間に　　　　　　　between meals

1日3回服用してください．

- Please take it three times a day.
  毎食前に　before each meal
  毎食後に　after each meal

毎回，2錠［包］服用してください．

- Please take two tablets [packets] each time.

粉薬はジュースやアイスクリームに混ぜてもいいです．

- You can mix this powder medicine with juice or ice cream.

その薬の効果は約3時間で切れるでしょう．

- The (effects of the) medicine will wear off in about three hours.

薬の効果が切れたら，また熱が出るかもしれません．

- Your fever might return once the effects of the medicine wear off.

この薬は効果がありませんでしたか？

- Did this medicine have any effect on you?
- Is this medicine working?
- Is this medicine not working?
- Is this medicine not helping?

薬は残っていますか？

- Do you have any medicine left (over)?
- Do you still have medicine?
- Are you out of medicine?
- Did you run out of medicine?

薬は何錠残っていますか？

- How many tablets are left over?
- How much medicine do you have left?

手持ちの薬がなくなってきていますか？

- Are you out of medicine?

患者：3錠だけ残っています．

- I have only three tablets left.
- There are only three tablets left.

患者：Aだけ残っています．

- Only A is left.

（薬の投与日数を増やしてほしいと言う患者さんには）

日本では，医師はこの薬を最大30日まで処方することが許可されています．

- In Japan, doctors are only permitted [allowed] to prescribe this medicine for a maximum of 30 days.

抗生物質（抗菌薬）は肺炎のリスクを下げるのに役立ちます．

- This antibiotic helps [will help] decrease the [your] risk of pneumonia.

咳の薬を処方します．

- I'll prescribe some pills for your cough.

その薬は咳［頭痛］をやわらげます．

- That medicine will help (with) your cough [headache].

この薬は頭痛［咳］によく効きます．

- This medicine 「works well [is good] for 「a headache [a cough].

頭痛を楽にするためにこの薬を飲んでください．

- Take this medicine to relieve your headache.
- Take this medicine for headache relief.

この薬は痛みをある程度やわらげます．

- This medicine will reduce [relieve] your pain to some extent.

この薬は痛みをかなりやわらげます．

- This medicine is very effective in reducing pain.

この薬は痛み止めとしても解熱薬としても効きます．

- This medicine works as both a pain-killer and an anti-pyretic.

頓服薬も出します．

- I'll prescribe some additional medicine that you can take as needed.

頭痛［熱，ひどい咳，発作など］があるときにのみ服用してください．

- Only take it when you have「a headache [a fever, a bad cough, an attack, etc.].

37.5度以上の発熱があるか，痛みが強いときに服用してください．

- You can [should] take it (only) if your temperature rises above 37.5 degrees or if you「have severe pain [are in a lot of pain].

次の頓服薬を飲むには最低6時間空けてください．

- You「have to [must] wait at least 6 hours before taking the next dose (of the additional medicine).
- You can take the additional medicine again after 6 hours.

胸痛があるとき，この薬を舌下してください．

- Please put this under your tongue when you have chest pain.
- Let this dissolve under your tongue when you have chest pain.

5分経っても胸痛があるときは，もう1錠追加してください．

- If you still have chest pain 5 minutes after the first dose, you can use one more tablet.

この薬を舌下する場合，座るか横になってください．

- When you put this under your tongue, you should (either) sit (down) or lie down.

便秘薬も出します．

- I'll prescribe a laxative as well.

この薬は便秘薬です．

- This (medicine) is a laxative.

睡眠薬の処方を書いておきます.

- I'll write a prescription for sleeping pills.

この薬を飲めば，気持ちが落ち着きます.

- This medicine will calm you down.
- This medicine will steady your nerves.

▶ 吸入・噴霧・点眼

この薬でよくならなければ，スプレー式の薬も使えます.

- If your condition doesn't improve with this medicine, you can use the spray-type (medicine) as well.

この吸入式の薬（アドエア®など）を1日2回使ってください．1回2目盛り分吸入してください．1回は［2目盛り分を］朝，あと1回は［さらに2目盛り分を］寝る前です.

- Use this inhaler twice a day. One dose is two puffs. Take 「one dose [two puffs] in the morning, and 「one dose [two more puffs] before you go to bed.

この薬（アラミスト®など）を1日1回，左右の鼻に2回ずつスプレーしてください.

- Spray twice into each nostril once a day.

この薬（フルナーゼ®など）を1日2回，左右の鼻に1回ずつスプレーしてください.

- Spray once into each nostril twice a day.

この目薬を1日4回，それぞれの目に1滴ずつ点眼してください.

- Apply one drop to each eye four times a day.

この目薬は目にしみるかもしれません.

- These eyedrops might (make your eyes) sting (a little).
- Your eyes might sting (a bit) from these eyedrops.

▶ 副作用

添付文書によると，（副作用として）約0.1%の人に頭痛が起こります．

- According to the (attached) directions, a headache occurs in about 0.1% of the patients (as a side effect).
- The accompanying directions say a headache occurs in about 0.1% of the patients.

もしかしたら副作用として吐き気が出るかもしれません．

- One possible side effect of this medicine is nausea.

この薬の短所として，眠気をもよおすかもしれません．

- The downside of this medicine is that it might [could] make you drowsy.

この薬の服用中は車を運転しないでください．

- Please don't drive while 「using this medicine [you are on this medicine].

それは初期にだけ生じることが多く，（慣れるにつれて）その後は次第になくなります．

- It usually happens only at the beginning, and then it disappears [goes away] gradually (as you get used to it).

慣らすために（この薬の）最小量から開始します．これにより副作用を少なくします．

- I will start you on [off with] the minimum dosage (of this medicine) so that you can get used to it first. This will reduce [minimize] the side effects.

次回はより多くの量を処方するつもりです．

- Next time I will prescribe you a higher dosage.

予防接種を受けているので，あなたは〜に対して免疫があると思います．

- You should be immune to 〜 since you were vaccinated.

自然感染のおかげで，あなたは〜に対して免疫があると思います．

- I believe you are now immune to 〜 since you had it before.

この冬，インフルエンザの予防接種を受けましたか？

- Did you get a flu shot this winter?
- Were you vaccinated against influenza this winter?

ワクチンの予約は受付でできます．

- You can schedule a date for your vaccination at the reception desk.
- You can make an appointment for your vaccination at the reception desk.

これは予防接種のスケジュールです．

- This is the vaccination schedule.

お子さんの母子手帳を見せてください．

- Please show me your child's maternity record [book].

お子さんには，11月10日に麻疹の予防接種をしましょう．

- Let's make an appointment for your child to get a measles vaccination on November 10th.

今日は〜の予防接種をします．

- I will give you a 〜 vaccine [vaccination] today.
- You can get a 〜 vaccination today.

お子さんをしっかり抱いていてください.

- **Please hold your child firmly.**

今日は激しい運動はしないでください.

- **Please don't exercise hard [strenuously] today.**

腕が少し腫れるかもしれません.

- **You might have slight swelling in your arm.**
- **Your arm might be slightly swollen.**

診断書〔Medical Certificate and Receipt〕p.156

診断書が必要ですか？

- Do you need a medical certificate?
- Do you need a written diagnosis?

今，診断書を書きます．受付で受け取ってください．

- I will write (up) your certificate (right now). You can 「get it [pick it up] at the reception desk (in a few minutes).

診断書は有料です．

- There is a charge for a medical certificate.
- We will (have to) charge you for a medical certificate.

診断書の費用には日本の通常の保険は適用されません．

- Japan's standard health insurance doesn't cover the cost of a medical certificate.

診断書には5,000円かかります．税抜きの価格ですよ．

- There is a 5,000 yen charge for a medical certificate. This doesn't include tax.
- The charge for a medical certificate is 5,000 yen. This doesn't include tax.
- There is a 5,000 yen charge for a medical certificate, plus tax.

それでよろしいでしょうか？

- Is that okay？
- Will that do？
- Will that work for you?

この書式でいいですか？

- Will this form [format] meet your needs?
- Will this form do [be okay]?

手書きかプリントされたものか，どちらがよいですか？

- Does the certificate need to be typed? Or is a hand-written one acceptable?

プリント版が必要な場合は，明日以降に受け取ることができます．

- If you need a typed certificate, you can pick it up tomorrow or anytime afterwards.
- If you need a typed certificate, it will be ready [available] tomorrow.

22 診察の終了

よくならなかったら，またお越しください.

- If you don't get [start feeling] better, please come (back) and see me again.

薬がなくなる前にお越しください.

- Please come (back) and see me before you run out of medicine.

無理をしないで2，3日後にまたお越しください.

- I want you to「take it easy [get some rest], then come back in a couple of days.

経過をみたいので今月23日にまたお越しください.

- Please come and see me on the 23rd of this month, as I'd like to know [check on]「your progress [how you're doing].
- Please come back on the 23rd of this month, as I'd like to follow up on your progress.

10月3日以降にお越しください.

- Please come back on October 3rd or any time after that.
- Please come back on the 3rd of October or any time after that.

いつでも都合のよいときにお越しください.

- Come (back) and see me whenever you like.

仕事は何時に終わりますか？

- What time do you leave from work?
- What time do you get off from [of] work?
- What time are you through [finished] with work?

6時までにこちら［クリニック］にお越しください.

- Be sure to get here [to my clinic] by 6 o'clock.

書類は次の土曜日にできているでしょう.

- The form will be ready this coming Saturday.
- The form will be ready on Saturday.

これで終わりです. 退出していいですよ.

- We are finished [done] (for) today. You are free to leave.

（患者さんが Thank you, doctor. とあいさつしたら）どういたしまして. お大事に.
さようなら.

- You are welcome. Take care. Good-bye.

23 会計とあいさつ

税込2,100円頂戴します.

- That comes to 2,100 yen including tax.
- That will be 2,100 yen including tax.
- 2,100 yen, please.

追加項目については1,000円の別料金をお支払いください.

- There is a surcharge of 1,000 yen for some additional items.

診断書の代金は5,000円＋税金になります.

- A medical certificate costs 5,000 yen + tax.
- You will be charged 5,000 yen + tax for a medical certificate.
- There is a charge of 5,000 yen + tax for a medical certificate.

おつりです.

- Here's your change.

（保険証と診察券を渡しながら）このクリニックにお越しの際は，いつも保険証と診察券を持参してください.

- From now on, when you visit this clinic, please bring your health insurance and registration cards.
- For all future visits, be sure to bring your health insurance and registration cards.

処方箋と領収書です.

- Here are your prescription and receipt.

どこの薬局でも処方箋の薬を調合してもらえます.

- You can have your prescription filled at any pharmacy.

お大事に！

- Take care of yourself!
- I hope you are feeling better soon!
- I hope you feel better soon!

24 他院への紹介・他院での精密検査

▶ 他院への紹介

ご希望であれば，他院を紹介できます．

- I can introduce you to another hospital if you want [like].

この治療で満足していなければ，他院を紹介しますよ．

- If you're not satisfied with this treatment, I'd be glad to introduce you to another hospital.

本日の［この］薬でよくならなければ，他院を紹介します．

- If today's [this] medicine doesn't work, I'd be glad to introduce you to another hospital.

診断がつかないので大学病院を紹介します．

- Let me introduce [refer] you to a university hospital since it is difficult [hard, tough] to diagnose your illness here.

木曜日の午前中に，私の紹介状を持ってその病院へ行ってください．

- Please go to the hospital on Thursday morning with my letter of introduction.

今，紹介状を書きます．

- I'll write a referral letter (right) now.

紹介状を忘れずに持っていってください．

- Don't forget to bring my letter of introduction (with you).

▶ 他院での精密検査

大学病院で精密検査を受けてください.

- I would like you to have [undergo] 「a complete physical examination [a detailed check-up, a detailed examination] at a university hospital.

頸の腫瘍について, 形成外科医に診てもらったほうがいいですよ.

- I recommend you see a plastic surgeon for your neck tumor.
- It'd be a good idea (for you) to see a plastic surgeon about your neck tumor.

他院へ行き腹部の CT［MRI］検査を受けてください.

- I would like you to go to another hospital to get 「a CT scan [an MRI] of your stomach.

CT 検査の予約をします.

- I will make an appointment for a CT scan.

CT 検査の日取りを決めましょう.

- Let's set [decide on] a date for your CT scan.
- Let's make an appointment for your CT scan.

いつがよろしいですか?

- When is it convenient for you?
- What would be a convenient date and time for you?

CT 検査は25日午後2時30分に始まります. 30分前には到着するようにしてください.

- Your CT scan will start at 2:30 p.m. on the 25th. Please 「get there [check in] at least 30 minutes before your scheduled time.

▶ 入退院

入院してください.

- You need to be admitted to the hospital.

- You need to be hospitalized.

入院してより手厚い治療を受けてください.

- You need to be hospitalized for more in-depth medical treatment.

しばらく入院する必要があります．詳しくは病院の医師に聞いてください.

- You need to be hospitalized for a while. The doctor at the hospital will give you more details.
- You need to be hospitalized for a while. For more details, consult with the doctor at the hospital.

おそらく約1週間で退院できるでしょう.

- It's possible you will「get out of [be discharged from, be released from] the hospital in about a week.

▶ 他院へのアクセス

X病院は厚木市のとなりの伊勢原市にあります.

- X Hospital is located in Isehara (City) next to Atsugi City.

電車で行きますか，車で行きますか？

- Will you go by train or car?
- Will you take a train or drive there?

電車を利用する場合

小田原行きの～線に乗って，C駅で降りてください.

- Take the ～ Line toward Odawara and get off at C Station.

小田原に向かって，Bの次の駅です.

- If you're heading toward Odawara, it's the station after B.

Aから2つ目の駅です.

- It's the second station from A.

駅はA，B，Cの順です.

- The station after A is B; the next station (after that) is C.

- The order of stations is A, B, and C.

路線バスを利用する場合

C駅北口の前でX病院行きの～バスに乗ることができます.

- You can catch [take, ride] the ～ bus for X Hospital in front of C Station's north exit.
- The ～ bus for X Hospital departs from C Station's north exit.

駅の近くで誰かにバス乗り場を尋ねてください.

- Ask somebody near the station where the bus stop is.
- If you can't find the bus stop, ask someone for help.

病院まで約10分かかります.

- It takes about 10 minutes to get to the hospital.
- It's about 10 minutes to the hospital (by bus).

病院の専用バスを利用する場合

その病院には患者さん用の無料シャトルバスがあります.

- The hospital has a free shuttle bus for patients.

東京駅から（無料の）シャトルバスを利用できます.

- There's a special shuttle bus you can take from Tokyo Station (free of charge).

バスは東京駅とX病院を往復しています.

- The only stops are Tokyo Station and X Hospital.
- A shuttle bus runs between Tokyo Station and X Hospital.
- A shuttle bus goes back and forth between Tokyo Station and X Hospital.

行き先はバスの前か横に書いてあります.

- The bus will have signage on the front or side indicating the final destination.
- The bus will have the final destination displayed somewhere on its front or side.

午前10時30分に腹部の CT 検査を予約してありますので，駅から9時45分のシャトルバスに乗るとよいでしょう．

- Since your CT scan appointment is at 10:30 a.m., I recommend you take the 9:45 shuttle bus from the station.

自動車を利用する場合

お車であれば，246号線を走ってください．

- If you're (planning on) driving, take Route 246.

病院は246号線沿いにあります．

- The hospital is on Route 246.
- The hospital is right off (of) Route 246.

ここから約15分かかります．

- It takes about 15 minutes to get there from here.

▶ 外　科

医師から

手術が必要です.

- You need to have「an operation [a surgical procedure done].

8月3日に入院となります. 手術は8月4日です.

- You'll「be hospitalized [check into the hospital] on August 3rd. The operation is on August 4th.

手術は局所麻酔で行います.

- The operation will be performed [done] using a local anesthetic.

手術は全身麻酔で行います.

- The operation will be performed [done] using a general anesthetic.
- We'll put you under general anesthesia.

(この手術での) 入院期間は通常約2週間です.

- Basically, you will be in the hospital for about two weeks.
- Patients undergoing this surgical procedure are normally hospitalized for about 2 weeks.

手術の合併症として, アレルギー反応, 出血, 感染があります.

- Possible complications from this surgery are allergic reactions, bleeding, and infection.

輸血が必要な場合があります.

- You might need a blood transfusion.

患者さんから

ここが痛いです.

- It hurts here.

まだ痛みがあります.

- I'm still in pain.

打ち身が痛みます.

- My [This] bruise is painful.

 bruise　[bruːz]

傷が痛みます.

- My wound [cut] hurts.
- My wound is painful.

右肩が痛みます.

- My right shoulder hurts.

膝が痛くてたまりません.

- My knee hurts in a bad way.
- My knee hurts a lot.
- My knee really hurts.
- My knee is killing me.
- I have severe pain in my knee.

 靴がきつくてたまらない.
My shoes are killing me.
My shoes are too tight; they hurt my feet.

左腕がしびれています.

- My left arm is numb.

昨日, 左腕がしびれました.

- My left arm went numb yesterday.

昨日から両下肢がしびれています.

- My legs have been numb since yesterday.

医師から

～が痛みますか?

- Do you have pain in your ～?

どこが痛みますか?

- Where does it hurt?

(ひどく)痛みますか?

- Does it hurt (a lot)?
- Is it painful?

私が押すと痛いですか?

- Does it hurt when I press on it?
- Does it hurt when I apply pressure?

(ひどく)腫れていますね.

- It's (badly) swollen.

いつけがをしたのですか?

- When did you get hurt?
- When did you hurt it?

どのようにしてけがをしたのですか?

- How did you get hurt?

転んだのですか?

- Did you fall down?

何かにぶつかりましたか?

- Did you bump [run] into something?

 bump into のほうが軽い衝突で, run into は強い衝突を連想させます.

何に頭をぶつけたのですか？

- What did you hit your head against [on]?

何に右肘をぶつけたのですか？

- What did you hit [> knock > bump] your right elbow against?

どこか他の部位を痛めましたか？

- Did you hurt any other part of your body?

右肩にけがをしていますか？

- Did you hurt your right shoulder?
- Does your right shoulder hurt?

肩こりがありますか？

- Do you have stiff shoulders?
- Are your shoulders stiff?

手のこわばりはありますか？

- Do you have stiff hands?
- Are your hands stiff?

坂を下るとき膝が痛みますか？

- Does your knee hurt when you walk downhill [downslope]?

坂を上るとき膝が痛みますか？

- Does your knee hurt when you walk uphill [upslope]?

足を引きずって歩きますか？

- Are you walking with a limp?
- Are you limping?
- Do you walk with a limp?
- Do you limp?

前屈してください.

- Bend forward.

後屈してください.

- Bend backward.

頚を後屈したとき腕に変化はありますか？

- Do you feel 「any changes [anything different] in your arm when you bend your neck backward?

かかとで歩いてください. ／かかと立ちしてください.

- Walk on your heels. ／Stand on your heels.

つま先で歩いてください. ／つま先立ちしてください.

- Walk on your tiptoes. ／Stand on your tiptoes.

診断・コメント

足首の捻挫ですね.

- I think you just [simply] sprained [twisted] your ankle.
- You have an ankle sprain.

骨は折れていません.

- Your bone is not fractured [broken].
- There's no (bone) fracture.

膝の軟骨が減って，痛みが出ているようです.

- Apparently your pain is due to a decrease in your knee cartilage.
- I think your knee hurts because it has very little cartilage.

膝の問題があるので，治るまでゴルフはお勧めしません.

- Because of your knee problem, I don't recommend you play golf until it heals.

この傷はじきに治るでしょう.

- Your wound will heal (up) soon.

この傷を治療する必要はありません.

- There's no need to treat the wound.

これは（治療しなくても）自然に治りますよ.

- This will [should] heal naturally (without any treatment).

自然に治るのを待ちましょう.

- Let it heal naturally.

この傷は思った以上に治るのに時間がかかるでしょう.

- This wound will probably take longer to heal than expected.

傷が深い［ひどい］ので，私には手当てできません.

- I cannot treat you for this laceration [wound, cut] because it is too deep [severe].

糖尿病患者の傷はすぐには治りません.

- Diabetic patients' wounds [cuts, lacerations] take a long time to heal.

パソコンを長時間使っていると首を痛めます.

- You will have neck problems if you use [operate] a personal computer for long hours.
- You'll have neck problems if you 「sit at [work on] your computer for 「too long [many hours].
- Using a computer many hours in a row can cause neck problems.

今症状がなくても，約2ヵ月は頭痛や吐き気，麻痺に気をつけてください. 慢性硬膜下血腫の可能性がありますので，この種の症状が出たらすぐに病院を受診してください.

- Even though you don't have any symptoms right now, you could develop headaches, nausea, and paralysis about two months from now. This would indicate that you likely have (a) chronic subdural hematoma. If you have these symptoms, go [get] to a hospital as soon as possible.

再　診

具合はいかがですか？

- How are you doing?
- How are you feeling?

～［肩，膝など］はどうですか？

- How is your ～[shoulder, knee, etc.] doing?

腫れはひきましたか？

- Has the swelling gone down?

（傷などが）よくなっています．

- It's improving.

（傷などが）よくなっていません．

- It's not improving.

切り傷はよくなっています．

- The cut is healing.

傷はまだ治っていません．

- The wound is [has] not yet healed.

傷が化膿しています．

- The wound has pus in it.
- The wound is discharging pus.
- The wound has pus coming out of it.

指の炎症が悪化しています．

- The inflammation in [of] your finger is getting worse.

薬を飲みましたが，まだよくなっていません．

- You've been taking the medicine, but your condition is still not improving.
- Your condition is still not improving even though you've been taking the medicine.

通常の細菌感染であれば，抗生物質（抗菌薬）は効いてきているはずです．

- If it were a typical bacterial infection, the antibiotic would be working by now.

治　療

この傷はなかなか治らないでしょう．

- This wound will take a long time to heal.

傷を縫う必要があります．

- You need stitches.

局所麻酔をして傷を縫います．

- Let me suture [sew up, stitch up] the wound [cut, laceration] using a local anesthesia.

消毒します．

- I'm applying [putting on] an antiseptic.

消毒薬が少ししみるかもしれません．

- It [The anti-septic] might sting a little.

局所麻酔をします．ちょっとちくっとします．

- I'm giving you a local anesthetic. You will feel a sting.

傷を3針縫いました．

- I put three stitches in the wound.
- I closed the wound with three stitches.

1週間後に糸［ホチキスの針］を取りましょう．

- I'll remove [take out] the stitches [staples] 「in a week [a week from today].

今日処方する消毒薬で傷を消毒してください．

- Use the anti-septic that I'm prescribing today to keep the wound disinfected.

シャワーは浴びてもいいですが，湯船には入らないでください．

- You can take a shower, but you should not take a bath.
- You can take a shower, but you should not submerge yourself in (the bathtub, water).

この傷から破傷風になるかもしれませんので，トキソイドを注射しておきましょう．

- You might [could] get tetanus from this [your wound], so I'll give you a tetanus shot today.

（痛みをやわらげるため）肩に湿布してください．

- Please put a medicated patch on your shoulder (for pain relief).

傷に絆創膏を貼ってください．

- Please apply a bandage to your wound [cut].
- Please put a bandage on your wound [cut].

包帯を足に巻きます．

- I will bandage (up) your foot.
- I will put a bandage on your foot.

足に包帯をしたほうがよいです．

- You need a bandage on your foot.

巻いたあと粘着テープで包帯をとめてください．

- Please fasten the bandage with adhesive tape after you roll it on.

下肢にギプスをあてなくてはなりません．

- You need to have [get] a cast on your leg.
- Your leg needs to be in a cast.
- We [I] need to put a cast on your leg.

松葉杖をついて歩く必要があります．

- You will need (to use) crutches.

医師から

麻酔担当の加藤です.

- Hello. I'm Dr. Kato, your anesthetist in charge.

あなたの手術の麻酔を担当します.

- I'll be giving [administering] you the anesthesia for your operation.

いくつかお尋ねします.

- I'd like to ask you some questions.

今まで麻酔薬のアレルギーはありましたか？

- Have you ever had an allergic reaction to any anesthetics?
- Do you have any allergies to anesthetics?

どんな反応でしたか？

- What kind of allergic reactions did you have?

ゆるんでいる歯はありますか？

- Do you have any loose teeth?

手術前に入れ歯, コンタクトレンズ, 指輪ははずしていただきます.

- You need to <u>take out</u> your dentures and contact lenses and also <u>take off</u> your ring before the operation.

 体の内部にある物をはずすときには take out, 外部（表面）にある物をはずすときには take off を使います.

明日の朝8:30に手術室に向かいます.

- You will [are scheduled to] leave here for the operation room at 8:30 tomorrow morning.

手術中はあなたのお世話をさせていただきます.

- I'll be looking after you during the operation.

（麻酔を）始める前に，マスクを通して酸素を吸っていただきます．

- Before we start, I'd like you to breathe some oxygen through [from] this mask.

体を酸素で満たすため，顔にマスクを付けます．

- I'll put this mask over your face to fill [flood] your body with oxygen.

リラックスして普通に呼吸してください．

- Just relax and breathe normally.

（手術が）終わりましたよ．

- We are (all) finished [done].

深呼吸して．

- Take deep breaths.

▶ 眼　科

患者さんから

だんだん視力が落ちてきています．

- My eyesight [vision] is deteriorating [getting worse].

目やにが出ます．

- I have a discharge coming from my eyes.
- I have pus coming out of my eyes.
- My eyes are discharging mucus.
- I have eye mucus.

眼精疲労があります．

- I have eyestrain.
- I have eye fatigue.
- My eyes are strained [fatigued].

右目のかすみがあるのです．

- My right vision is blurry.

- I have blurred vision in my right eye.

ときどき目が痛みます.
- I sometimes feel pain in my eyes.
- My eyes hurt sometimes.

目がかゆいです.
- My eyes itch.
- My eyes feel itchy.
- I have itchy eyes.

医師から

コンタクトレンズをしていますか？
- Do you wear contact lenses?

すみずみまではっきり見えますか？
- Is your vision perfect?

目のかすみはありますか？
- Is your vision blurry?

左目がぼやけて見えますか？
- Do you have blurred vision in your left eye?

物が二重に見えますか？
- Are you seeing double?
- Do you see two of everything?
- Do you have double vision?

眼底検査

目薬を使って瞳孔を開き，目の中を観察します.

- To examine the back of your eyes, I'm going to use these eyedrops to dilate the pupils.
- These eyedrops are for checking the inner part of your eyes by looking through the pupils.

- These eyedrops are used to check your eyes; they allow me to see through your pupils.

少しの間，待合室でお待ちください．

- Please wait in the waiting room for a little bit.

 for a while は長く待たせる感じになるので，ここでは for a little bit.

呼ばれるまでここにいてください．

- Please wait here until I call your name.
- Please wait here. We'll let you know when to come in.

（頭が固定されるよう）あごを台に乗せて，おでこを器具にしっかりと付けてください．

- Please put your chin and your forehead firmly on the support (to keep your head steady).

少しの間，まばたきしないでください．はい，もうまばたきしていいです．

- 「Don't blink [Try not to blink] for a little bit. OK. You can blink now.

目薬のせいでまぶしく見えるので，数時間は普通に歩くこと，車を運転することができません．

- These eye drops will make your eyes sensitive to light, so you won't be able to walk or drive normally for a few hours.

瞳孔が開いているので，このあと3時間車の運転をしないでください．

- （点眼前）These eyedrops will dilate your pupils, so please don't drive for the next three hours.
- （点眼後）The pupils of your eyes are now dilated, so please don't drive for the next three hours.

眼圧検査
空気が出て目に当たります．大きく目を開けてください．

- I'm going to shoot a puff of air into your eyes. Please keep your eyes open wide.

診断・コメント

視力はよいです.

- You have good eyesight [vision].
- Your eyesight [vision] is good [excellent, normal].

視力がわるいです.

- You have poor eyesight [vision].

右目の視力が弱いです.

- You have poor vision in your right eye.

近視です.

- You are near-sighted.

遠視です.

- You are far-sighted.

乱視です.

- You are astigmatic.

 astigmatic　[æstɪgmǽtɪk]

老眼です. 加齢によるものです.

- You are far-sighted. This is common as you get older.

老眼鏡を使ったほうがいいです.

- You need reading glasses.
- You should get [use] reading glasses.

眼鏡をかけたほうがいいです. 早めに眼鏡屋さんに行くことをおすすめします.

- You need glasses. I recommend you see an optician as soon as possible.

 you go to an optician's shop というよりも you see an optician が普通.

視野が狭いです.

- You have a limited field [range] of vision.
- Your field of vision is limited.

失明するかもしれません.

- (There is a possibility that) you may lose your eyesight.
- You may go blind.

治　療

この目薬を1日3回点眼してください. 1回1滴または2滴さしてください.

- Use these eye drops three times a day. Put one or two drops each time.

この目薬は少ししみます.

- These eye-drops might sting (your eyes) a little.
- Your eyes might sting when you use these eye-drops.

▶ 耳鼻咽喉科

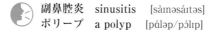

副鼻腔炎　sinusitis　[sàɪnəsáɪtəs]
ポリープ　a polyp　[páləp/pɔ́lɪp]

患者さんから

くしゃみ

くしゃみが（たくさん）出ます.

- I am sneezing (a lot).

くしゃみをこらえることができません.

- I cannot stop sneezing.

鼻水

鼻水が出ます.

- I have a runny nose.
- My nose is running.
- I have nasal drip.

鼻水が黄色です.

- I have yellow (nasal) mucus.
- My nose is discharging yellow mucus.
- My (nasal) mucus is yellow.

鼻づまり

鼻づまりがあります.

- My nose is (all) stuffed up.

 all を入れると「すっかり」の意.

- My nose is stuffy [congested].
- I have a stuffy nose.
- My nasal passages are blocked.
- I have nasal congestion.

鼻くそでいっぱいです.

- My nose is filled with dry [dried] mucus.

鼻声

鼻声になっています.

- I have a nasal voice.

嗄声

声がかれています.

- My voice is hoarse.

声が出なくなっています.

- I've lost my voice.
- I have laryngitis.

喉の痛み

喉が痛みます.

- I have a sore throat.

- My throat is sore.

喉がヒリヒリ［イガイガ］します.

- My throat feels irritated.

鼻をほじる
何度も鼻をほじりました.

- I scratched the inside of my nose a lot.
- I've been scratching the inside of my nose a lot.

鼻をかむ
鼻をかんでもいいですか？

- May I blow my nose?
- Is it okay if I blow my nose?

鼻血
鼻血が出ています.

- My nose is bleeding.
- I have a nosebleed.

昨晩, たくさん鼻血が出ました.

- I had a severe nosebleed last night.
- My nose was bleeding a lot last night.

嗅覚障害
においがほとんどわかりません.

- I can hardly smell anything.
- I'm losing my sense of smell.

耳垢
両耳が耳垢でいっぱいでしょうか.

- I wonder if my ears are full of wax.
- I wonder if I have a lot of wax in my ears.

耳漏

耳から液が出ます.

- I have a discharge of fluid from my ear.
- My ear is discharging fluid.
- There is fluid coming out of my ear.

耳痛

右耳が痛みます.

- My right ear aches.
- I have pain in my right ear.
- I have an earache in my right ear.

耳鳴

耳鳴りがします.

- I have ringing in my ears.
- My ears are ringing.
- I have tinnitus.

 tinnitus　[tínətəs/tənáɪtəs]

難聴

耳の聞こえがわるいです.

- I am hard of hearing.
- My hearing is bad [poor, not so good].
- I can't hear very well.
- I have difficulty hearing.

右耳が聞こえなくなりました.

- I've lost my hearing in my right ear.
- I can't hear (anything) in my right ear.

めまい

ふらふらします.

- I feel lightheaded.
- I feel dizzy.

部屋が回転しているように感じました.

- I felt like the room was spinning.

回転性のめまいがします.

- I have [am suffering from] vertigo.
- My balance is off.

頭がグラグラします.

- My head is spinning.

空腹［熱，疲労］で失神しそうです.

- I feel faint from hunger [the heat, exhaustion].

ふわふわ浮いている感じです.

- I feel like [as if] I'm floating.

医師から

両耳が耳垢でいっぱいです.

- Your ears are full of wax.
- You have wax in your ears.

耳垢をとりますよ.

- Let me remove your earwax.
- Let's remove that earwax.
- Let's get that earwax out.

耳から液が出ていますよ.

- You have a discharge of fluid from your ear.
- Your ear is discharging fluid.

鼻くそでいっぱいですよ.

- Your nose is filled with dry [dried] mucus.

鼻くそをとりますよ.

- Let me remove your dry [dried] mucus.

鼻に出血した痕があります.

- There are traces of dried blood inside your nose.

 traces of 〜は「微量の〜」の意をもつ.

鼻を強くほじらないでください.

- Don't scratch the inside of your nose so hard.

 pick your nose は鼻くそを取り除く行為で大人げないイメージがあるので, ここでは避けたほうがよいでしょう.

においがわかりますか？

- Do you have a problem with your sense of smell?
- Do you have a smell disorder?

扁桃腺が腫れていて膿を出しています.

- Your tonsils are swollen and discharging pus.

喉に後鼻漏を認めます.

- I can see post-nasal drip in your throat.

声帯を休めるために, ささやく話し方をしてください.

- Please whisper [speak softly] to rest your vocal cords.

聴力検査

聴力検査を受けていただきたいです.

- I'd like you to get a hearing test.
- I'd like you to get your hearing tested.
- Let's get your hearing tested.

このヘッドホンを付けてください.

- Please put on these headphones.

何か聞こえたらボタンを押してください.

- Press the button when you hear something.

何か聞こえている間はボタンを押し続けてください.

- Hold down the button as long as you can hear something.
- Continue to hold down the button until you can't hear anything.
- Release the button when the sound stops.

いい聴力です.

- Your hearing is normal [good].

聴力に問題はありません.

- There is nothing wrong with your hearing.

▶ 皮膚科

患者さんから

首にたくさんの発疹ができました.

- I have a rash on my neck.
- My neck (area) broke out in a rash.

体中に（ひどい）発疹が広がりました.

- I broke out in a (terrible) rash.
- I have a rash all over my body.
- A rash broke out over my whole body.
- A rash broke out all over my body.

背中が痒いです.

- My back itches.
- My back is itchy.

スズメバチが私の顔を刺しました.

- A wasp stung me on my face.
- I got stung by a wasp on my face.

皮膚がガサガサしています．

- **I have rough skin.**
- **My skin is scaly.**

単純疱疹　herpes simplex, simple herpes
　口唇ヘルペス　labial herpes, cold sore

 labial　[léɪbiəl]

 herpes　[hə́ːrpiːz]

　性器ヘルペス　genital herpes
帯状疱疹　herpes zoster, shingles
蕁麻疹　hives
梅毒　syphilis
虫刺され　an insect bite
真菌症　a fungal infection [disease]
　真菌　fungus
　　白癬菌　ringworm
　　カンジダ　candida
足白癬（いわゆる水虫）　athlete's foot =foot fungus
爪白癬（いわゆる爪水虫）　fungal nail disease
脱毛症　alopecia=hair loss

 alopecia　[æ̀ləpíːʃə]

an eruption　発疹
a spot　斑点，まだら，しみ，吹き出物，ほくろ
a mole　ほくろ
a pimple　にきび

 acne は「にきび」という病名で，不可算名詞．

 acne　[ǽkni]

a boil　おでき
a swelling　腫れもの
a wart　いぼ

 wart　[wɔ́ːrt]

a canker=a mouth ulcer　アフタ性口内炎

 日本語でいうアフタ an aphtha (>aphthae) は日常英会話では使われない．

a rash　多数の赤いポツポツ

 単数でも病態を指す．病名に近い．heat rash は「あせも」という病名．

a blister　水疱
a bump　こぶ（打撲時の内出血）
a lump　しこり（小さめ）
a mass　しこり（大きめ）

138

踵がひび割れています.

- My heels are chapped.

頭に（少し）フケが出ます.

- I have (a little) dandruff.

髪が薄くなってきています.

- I'm losing my hair.

髪が抜けてきています.

- My hair is falling [coming] out.

（強い）体臭があります.

- I have (strong) body odor.

 odor [óʊdər]

腋臭があります.

- I have underarm odor.

医師から

どこが痒いですか？

- Where does it itch?
- Where do you feel itchy?
- Where do you itch?
- What part itches?

背中が痒いですか？

- Does your back itch?
- Does your back feel itchy?

体中が痒いですか？

- Do you feel itchy all over?
- Do you itch all over?

足の指の間が（ひどく）痒いですか？

- Does it feel (especially) itchy between your toes?

つい，掻いてしまうのですね？

- Do you scratch「without thinking [unconsciously]?
- Do you unconsciously scratch yourself?

痒い場所を掻かないように．

- Don't scratch where it itches.

いつ皮膚の異常に気づきましたか？

- When did you realize [notice] you had a skin problem?

いつポツポツが首に出ましたか？

- When did the rash「break out [appear] on your neck?
- When did you get that rash on your neck?

前腕が何かに触れましたか？ それとも前腕に何かを付けましたか？

- Did your forearm come into contact with anything? Or did you put anything on your forearm?

新しい石鹸に変えましたか？

- Did you change to a new soap?

蜂に刺されましたか？

- Were you stung by a bee?

皮膚を顕微鏡で調べさせてください．

- Let me examine a sample of your skin under a microscope.
- Let's take a skin sample and do a biopsy.

顕微鏡検査用に皮膚標本を採らせてください．

- Let's take a biopsy of your skin.

結果が出るまで約40分かかります．

- It will take about 40 minutes to get the results.
- We'll know the results in about 40 minutes.

• We should know the results in about 40 minutes.

明日結果が出るので，再度お越しください．

　　• We'll know the results tomorrow; (so) come back and see me then.

パッチを鶏眼［胼胝］に4日間貼ったままにしてください．

　　• Please keep [leave] the patch on your corn [callus] for four days.

診断・コメント

これは自然に治りますよ．

　　• This will heal (up) naturally without any treatment.

この発疹はそのままにしておきましょう．

　　• Try to leave the rash alone.
　　• Let it heal on its own.

この問題は〜［毛染め，日光，ストレス］と関係があるようです．

　　• This problem seems to be related to 〜 [hair dye, sunlight, stress].

再　診

（傷，発疹などは）どうなっていますか？

　　• How is it going?

　　患者：よくなっています．／よくなっていません．

　　　　• It's improving.／It's not improving.

腫れはひきましたか？

　　• Has the swelling gone down?

通常の細菌感染であれば，抗生物質（抗菌薬）を飲んでいるので，よくなっているはずです．

　　• If you have a typical bacterial infection, it should heal with no problem since you are taking an antibiotic.

治　療

腕に軟膏を塗り込んでください.

- You need to apply [put, rub, dab] the ointment on your arms.

この軟膏を塗っても治りません.

- This won't get better using this ointment.
- This will not heal (up) using this ointment.

薬だけ飲んだとしてもよくならないでしょう.

- This likely won't heal by taking oral medicine alone.

爪水虫は，薬を飲まないと治りません.

- A fungal nail disease won't heal unless you take an oral medicine.

膿を出すために小さな針で皮膚を刺さなくてはなりません. そうしなければ痛みが続くでしょうし，回復が遅れるでしょう.

- I will have to prick your skin with a small needle to release the pus, otherwise your pain will continue and healing will take longer.

この腫瘍は切除しましょう.

- Let's remove this tumor.

この腫瘍はレーザーで焼きましょう.

- Let's burn off this tumor with a laser beam.

心配しないでください，局所麻酔を使いますから，痛くないですよ.

- Don't worry, I'll use a local anesthetic, so it won't hurt.

同意していただけますか？

- Do [May] I have your consent [permission] to do this?
- Do [May] I have your permission to proceed?
- Will you give me your consent to do this?

患者から

やけどをしてしまいました．

- I burned myself.

マッチ［やかん，バーベキュー網，オーブンドア，熱い平鍋など］で，指をやけどしてしまいました．

- I burned my finger on [with] the match [the kettle, the barbecue grill, the oven door, the hot pan, etc.].

※熱傷の原因が蒸気もしくは熱い液体の場合

上記 burn の代わりに scald を使います．

- I scalded myself.
- I scalded my finger on [with] the steam [the hot water, the kettle water, the hot oil, etc.].

また，この場合，熱傷の原因を主語にして表現することも可能です．

- The steam scalded me on my finger.
- The hot coffee scalded my tongue.

 しかしながら，最近の若い人では burn と scald を原因から区別して使うとは限らなくなってきています．

診断とコメント

やけどは3つの重症度に分類されます．あなたはⅡ度熱傷です．

- Burns [Scalds] are classified into three categories. You have a second-degree burn [scald].

このやけどは瘢痕を残す可能性があります．

- My guess is (that) this burn will leave a scar.
- This burn will probably [most likely] leave a scar.

治　療

水疱は今日はそのままにしておきましょう．

- Let's leave the blister alone today.
- Let's not remove the blister today.

 leave 〜 alone は熟語で，「かまわずそのままにしておく」の意味です．

水疱はすでに破れているので取り除きます．

- I'll remove the blister since it has already ruptured.

ハイドロコロイドなど湿潤療法

①このパッチはこのまま最大7日間貼ったままにしてください．

- You should keep [leave] this patch intact [as it is, untouched, on your skin] for「at most [not more than] 7 days.

②白い部分が端まできたら，傷からパッチをとり，取り替えてください．

- When the white area spreads to the edge of the patch, remove it from the burn, then replace the patch.

▶ **泌尿器科**

医師から

1日何回排尿しますか？

- How many times a day do you urinate?

排尿の間隔はどのくらいですか？

- What is the interval [amount] of time between each urination?

睡眠中は排尿で何回目が覚めますか？

- How many times do you wake up at night to urinate?

頻尿がありますか？

- Do you experience frequent urination?
- Do you urinate frequently?

どのくらい頻回ですか？ たとえば10分毎とか，1時間毎とか．

- How frequently? For example, every ten minutes or every hour.

尿が出しにくいことはありますか？

- Is it sometimes difficult for you to start urinating?
- Do you have difficulty starting to urinate?

排尿に時間がかかりますか？

- Does it take more time to urinate than it did before?
- Do you spend more time urinating than before?

尿の勢いが弱いですか？

- Is your urine stream weak?

尿線は細いですか？

- Is your urine stream narrow?
- Do you have a narrow urine stream?

残尿感はありますか？

- Do you feel like your bladder is not empty even after urination?

尿をもらすことがありますか？

- Do you ever leak urine?

排尿中に痛みを感じますか？

- Do you feel any pain during urination?
- Do you feel any pain when you urinate?

痛みは尿の出口ですか？ それとも下腹部ですか？

- Is the pain around [in] the area of the urethral opening? Or (is it) in the lower abdomen?

血尿が出ましたか？

- Was there blood in your urine?
- Have you noticed blood in your urine?

ペニスから膿あるいは透明な分泌物が出ますか？

- Is your penis secreting pus or a clear discharge?
- Do you have any discharge from your penis?

多量の水を飲んで改善する膀胱炎もあります．

- In some cases, cystitis [UTI] gets better just by drinking lots of water.

前立腺を調べるために直腸に指を入れます.

- I'll have to insert my finger into your rectum to examine your prostate.

左を下にして横を向いて膝を抱えてください.

- Please lie on your left side with your knees up.

▶ 産　科

患者さんから

予定より1週間以上生理が遅れています.

- My period is more than a week late.

数ヵ月生理がこないので, 妊娠したかもしれません.

- I haven't gotten my period for a few months, so I ⌈might be [think I'm] pregnant.

妊娠3ヵ月です.

- I'm three months pregnant.
- I'm in the [my] third month (of pregnancy).

つわりがひどいのです.

- I have severe [really bad] morning sickness.

妊娠8週で流産しました.

- I had a miscarriage in my 8th week of pregnancy.

中絶しました.

- I had [got] an abortion.

中絶したいのです.

- I decided to have [get] an abortion.
- I've decided to terminate my pregnancy.
- I want to get an abortion.

子供ができないのです.

- I'm sterile [infertile].
- I can't have children.

避妊薬を服用したいです.

- I'd like to take (oral) contraceptives.
- I'd like to take birth-control pills.

ピルを服用しています.

- I'm on the pill.

医師から

ご自分で妊娠診断キットを使いましたか？

- Did you test yourself with a pregnancy test kit?

尿で妊娠検査をしましょう.

- Let's test your urine to see if you're pregnant.
- Let's do a pregnancy test. I'll need a sample of your urine.

あなたは妊娠しています.

- You are pregnant.

つわりはありますか？

- Do you have morning sickness?

妊娠何週ですか？

- How many weeks pregnant are you (now)?

今まで流産したことはありますか？

- Have you ever had any miscarriages?

あなたは妊娠6週です.

- You are six weeks pregnant.
- You are in the sixth week of pregnancy.

出産はいつですか？

- When are you supposed to give birth?
- When are you expecting (your baby)?
- When is your baby due?

予定日は4月9日です．

- Your baby is due on April 9th.
- Your due date is April 9th.

赤ちゃんは順調に育っています．

- Your baby is growing [progressing] normally.

経腟分娩でしたか，それとも帝王切開でしたか？

- Did you have a vaginal delivery or a Cesarean section?

帝王切開になるかもしれません．

- You might need a Cesarean section.
- The doctor might have to deliver your baby by Cesarean section.

本来，妊娠中は薬を飲まないほうがよいです．

- Basically, it's better not to take medication during pregnancy.

特に妊娠15週までは薬を飲むのを控えたほうがよいでしょう．

- You should especially refrain from taking any medication until the 15th week of pregnancy.

今日はより安全で弱めのお薬を最小量で処方します．

- Today I'll prescribe you a much safer and milder medicine at a minimum dosage.

体重は増えすぎないように注意してください．

- Be careful not to gain too much weight.

性行為はしばらく控えてください．

- Please refrain from sexual activities for a while.

どこで分娩しますか？

- Where do you want to give birth to your baby?
- Where do you want to have your baby?

✚ **分娩に関する表現**

痛みの間隔は？10分間隔ですか？

- How often do you feel pain? Every ten minutes?

痛みは毎回どのくらい続きますか？

- How long does the pain last each time?

破水しましたか？

- Has your water broken?

赤ちゃんはあと6時間くらいで産まれるでしょう．

- Your baby will be born in about six hours.

頑張って！

- Hang in there!

いきんで！

- Push hard!

▶ **婦人科**

患者さんから

生理が不規則です．

- My menstrual cycle is irregular.

毎月，生理痛がひどいです．

- I have severe 「menstrual pain [cramps]」 every month.

先週，不正出血がありました．

- Last week I had unexpected vaginal bleeding.

陰部にできものがあります.

- I have a boil [swelling] on my genitals.

陰部が痒いです.

- My genitals itch.
- My genitals are itchy.

陰部が痛いです.

- I have pain in my genitals.
- My genitals hurt.

医師から

生理痛はありますか？

- Do you have menstrual cramps?
- Is your period painful?

生理中ですか？

- Are you having your (menstrual) period?
- Are you menstruating?

生理は規則的ですか？

- Are your periods regular?

最後の生理はいつでしたか？

- When did you last have your period?

最後の生理の始まりはいつでしたか？

- When did your period last start?
- What was the first day of your last period?

最後の生理の終わりはいつでしたか？

- When did your period last end?
- What was the last day of your most recent period?

まだ生理はありますか？

- Do you still have your period?

生理が止まりましたか？

- Did you go through menopause yet?

更年期ですか？

- Are you going through menopause?

急に顔がほてりますか？

- Do your hot flashes come on suddenly?

ホットフラッシュや発汗，動悸などの症状はありますか？

- Do you have any symptoms such as hot flashes, sweating, or palpitations?

腟からおりものが出ますか？

- Do you have vaginal discharge?
- 「Do you have [Are you having] any discharge from your vagina?

陰部が痒いですか？

- Do your genitals itch?
- Does your genital area itch?

陰部に水疱があります．

- You have blisters on your genitals.

指を入れて内診します．

- I'm going to insert my finger into your vagina to do an internal examination.
- I'll do an internal examination (by inserting my finger into your vagina).

腟鏡診をします．

- I'm going to give you an examination using a speculum [specular device].

医師から

お子さんはどうしましたか？

- What is your child's (health) issue?

母子手帳を見せてください．

- Please show me the maternity record (book) of your child.

お子さんは妊娠何週で生まれましたか？

- How many weeks were you pregnant when your child was born?

お子さんの生まれたときの体重はいくらでしたか？

- How much did your child weigh at birth?

授乳中ですか？

- Are you breast-feeding?

1日何回ミルクを与えますか？

- How many times do you feed him [her] each day?

ミルクの飲みは普通ですか？

- Does your child drink milk normally?

人工乳で育てていますか？

- Are you bottle-feeding?

毎回どのくらい人工乳を飲みますか？

- How much formula milk does your child drink at feeding time?

すでに固形食［離乳食］を開始しましたか？

- Have you started him [her] on 「solid food [baby food] yet?

お子さんは簡単な言葉を話しますか？

- Does your child say simple words now?
- Does your child talk a little now?

Medical Fee Policy

To All Patients:

This clinic offers medical treatment to all patients with or without health insurance.

Patients with health insurance coverage must pay 10%–30% in cash for medical services at this clinic.

Patients without health insurance coverage will be required to pay the full amount for medical services rendered. The cost may vary from _____ yen + tax to _____ yen + tax for routine examinations and treatment.

Those with overseas traveler's medical insurance coverage will be required to pay the entire sum in cash upfront. Patients are responsible for filing for reimbursement with their insurance company.

If a standard medical check-up is required by your school or company, the expenses are not covered by health insurance. The fee will be approximately _____ yen.

The charge for a medical certificate is _____ yen + tax.

Prescription medicine costs are not included, as they must be purchased from a pharmacy. For all other necessary items or services, you will be informed in advance of the cost.

We do not accept credit cards. All payments must be made in full at time of consultation.

If you understand and agree to the conditions above, please fill out the questionnaire and wait in the waiting room until your name is called.

Medical Questionnaire

First Name		Date of Birth	Month	Day	Year
Family Name					
Address		Sex	Male	Female	
		Home Country			
Telephone	① — —	Occupation			
	② — —				

1. What is your medical issue?

What are your symptoms? _____

If it's an injury, how did it happen? _____

When did it start? _____

Any other reason to visit this office? _____

2. Have you ever had any special disorders?

(Examples : Bronchial Asthma, Hypertension, Hyperlipidemia, Gout (Hyperuric Acidemia), Diabetes, Heart Disease, Liver Disease, Kidney Disease, Brain Disease, Sinusitis, Appendicitis, Atopic Dermatitis, Allergic Rhinitis, etc.)

No / Yes ⇒ ① _____ When? _____

② _____ When? _____

③ _____ When? _____

④ _____ When? _____

⑤ _____ When? _____

154

3. Are you under a doctor's care for anything?

No / Yes ⇒ _____

4. Are you taking any medicine?

No / Yes ⇒ _____

5. Are you allergic to anything?

No / Yes ⇒ _____ (Reaction = _____)

6. Alcohol?

No / Occasionally / Everyday

_____ days per week

Beer _____ Glass

Japanese Sake _____ Sake Bottle

Whiskey _____ Can

Wine _____ Bottle

7. Do you smoke?

No / Yes ⇒ _____ cigarettes per day

8. Do you know of any serious or chronic illnesses in your family?

No / Yes ⇒ _____

9. Are you pregnant? (Female only)

No / Yes ⇒ How many weeks/months? _____

10. Are you breast-feeding?

No / Yes

155

Medical Certificate and Receipt

Patient's name				Patient's Date of Birth		/	/
Date of illness (first symptom) or injury	/	/		Any other disease affecting present condition		No	Yes
Date of first consultation	/	/		Is condition due to pregnancy?		No	Yes
Has patient ever had same or similar symptoms?	No	Yes		If yes, give approx. date		/	/
				If yes, did patient receive any treatment for prior symptoms by any doctor?		No	Yes
Period of your treatment	Outpatient			Date: / / ~ / /			
Diagnosis or nature of illness or injury							
Date of Recovery	/	/		Prognosis (in case of injury)		Good	Poor

Date / /

○○ **Clinic**

(Address of the clinic)

Tel: +81-○○-○○○-○○○○

Attending Physician: Dr.

Signature:

_____

Procedures, medical services or supplies furnished	Charges	Date of service
Management		
Tests		

Issue
  Prescription
  Introduction Letter
  Medical Certificate		

Others		
TOTAL CHARGE		
Amount paid		
Balance due		

memo

memo

memo

memo

memo

謝　辞

この本の出版に際して，ニューヨークで medical scribe として活躍している Grady　Sullivan 氏にはより native な表現に関して助言をいただいたこと，南山堂の古川晶彦氏，小枝克寿氏をはじめとするスタッフには企画・編集で多大なご苦労をしていただいたことに対し，深く感謝申し上げます．

―――― 著者略歴 ――――

加藤 秀一

かとうクリニック（内科・アレルギー科・麻酔科）院長
医学博士

神奈川県横浜市出身
1981 年　岩手医科大学医学部卒業
1996 年　東海大学医学部講師
1997 年　英国 GENERAL MEDICAL COUNCIL に MEDICAL
　　　　PRACTITIONER 登録し，Gloucestershire Royal Hospital にて臨床およ
　　　　び研究に従事
1999 年　かとうクリニックを開院．現在に至る

Timothy M. Sullivan

ビジネスコンサルタント
翻訳家

アメリカ合衆国シカゴ出身
1985 年　国際基督教大学（異文化コミュニケーション）を卒業
　　　　し，英会話教師，英文リライター
1987 年　異文化マネージメントの架け橋となるべく，調整役・
　　　　通訳としてアメリカおよび日本の企業に従事
2003 年　「これで海外工場でうまく仕事ができる－使える工場英語＆知っておく
　　　　べきビジネス・カルチャー」（PHP 出版）を出版
2019 年　日本に拠点を置き活動中

すぐに使える診療英語

2020 年 4 月 1 日　1 版 1 刷　　　　　　　　　　©2020
2022 年 4 月 20 日　　　2 刷

著　者
加藤秀一　Timothy M. Sullivan
（かとうひでかず）

発行者
株式会社 南山堂　代表者 鈴木幹太
〒113-0034　東京都文京区湯島 4-1-11
TEL 代表 03-5689-7850　www.nanzando.com

ISBN 978-4-525-02241-9

A0224120102-A